'This new book by Nathan Szajnberg, a child psychiatrist, researcher, says, "this is a personal book." It retells tales of his many returns to Israel to study children and families at the Israeli-Gaza border following the October 7th terrorist attack and displaced children from Ethiopia and IDF soldiers. His tale is likened to a "descent into hell." The author is our Virgil, asking us to attend with a Solomonic "listening heart" to the pain and terror described—that also references his personal story of his father's miraculous rescue from death at Auschwitz and his own birth at a Displaced Persons Camp. As, in the Inferno, the descent is a necessary mid-life trial—preceding repair and transformation. For Szajnberg it is a calling to listen at the side of the victims as they "grieve and hope" or long for hostages' return. It documents children's synthetic capacities to inject hope while assimilating trauma. In short Szajnberg's felt "call" is part of a transformative participation—reminding the reader to remember before we are fully fit to move forward constructively.'

Theodore Shapiro, MD, *Emeritus Professor of Psychiatry,*
Weill Cornell Medicine, Editor of
Journal of Psychoanalytic Association, *1982–1993*

'A much-needed perspective with moving appeals of human suffering.
How to recover from being in Hell, especially when many of your beloveds were slaughtered there?

This book explores this question after meeting with evacuated children, parents, those whose friends and relatives were murdered or are being held hostage. The book also addresses the acute stress disorder of soldiers and how to treat them in a war zone. We hear from physicians and nurses who must carry on their clinical responsibilities even as their sons and daughters are in combat, even as they themselves are under bombardment. The author, born in an American Displaced Persons Camp in Germany, felt a responsibility to the Jewish people and State, given that his father was in Auschwitz and was ultimately saved by Allied troops. When sitting with IDF physician-officers, he knew that they were risking their lives to rescue Israeli hostages. His obligation was to help them as much as he could and bring the stories of the children, parents and soldiers to us. The author seeks and calls for the rebuilding of wounded lives and communities.'

Michael Eigen, *Author of* The Psychotic Core, Faith, Emotional Storm, *and* Bits of Psyche

'This extraordinary book, an unusual integration of historical analysis, subjective experience and interpreted myth, represents the author's shock over the hell of October 7th savage assault on Israel, its willful repetition of the structure of the Holocaust, and its enactment of hell as a human reality, starting from his father's experience of Auschwitz, Szajnberg explores the descent into hell by the heroes of the three great myths of Dante's Inferno, Odyssey's descent to the underworld, and Anaeus drive through hell. The satanic features of hell, the sadistic rapes and murder of women, the cruel torture and murder of infants and children, the joyful, savage sadistic attacks of the Hamas assailants of October 7th merge nationally with the mythic hells.

Szajnberg connects October 7th developments with his father's multiple experiences of dread for his life, the anxious despair of father trying to survive, and generalized this effort to the task of survivor in contemporary sadistically authoritarian regimes.

These observations of horror lead into the problem of witness: how to listen without contamination by despair and hatred? Again, the author links the answer to this question to his personal efforts to travel to Israel to support the victims, witnesses and all those affected by the Hamas assault with the general action of the country to protect children and families from the assault on their personality and self-esteem. Szajnberg describes the massive efforts to provide opportunities by multiple organizations supporting a broad spectrum of children and affected population groups, visitors and others and the Israeli solders' contribution to treating post-traumatic stress disorders. The illustrations of the healing potential of traumatized children's psychotherapy are a meaningful concluding subject of this book.

In this volume, full of information about hell on earth and how to deal with its consequences effectively, an underlying theme is the very fact of the permanent risk of outbreak of hell underneath the apparently dominant surface of good will and understanding, love and human kindness. Freud's "Civilization and its Discontents," his basic drive theory of libido and aggression, emerge as a fundamental condition of human existence. And the need to combat hell and heal the survivors are basic human tasks. This volume focuses on the healing process but reminds us of the inevitable recurrence of hell, even in its relatively localized threat by Hamas.'

Otto F. Kernberg, MD, *Professor Emeritus,*
Weill Cornell Medical College, Training and Supervising Analyst,
Columbia University Psychoanalytic Center for Training and Research

War Trauma

How to work with those traumatized in war? Read this book.

Following the events of October 7, the author explores work in Israel with traumatized children, parents, communities, and soldiers. He offers guidance for working with civilian and military patients after wartime murder, rape, kidnapping, and displacement. See the children's drawings and listen to their stories as well as those of evacuated parents and battle-worn soldiers.

This deeply compassionate and informed approach is key reading for psychoanalysts, psychotherapists, and others during and after war.

Nathan Moses Szajnberg, MD, was born in a Displaced Persons Camp and grew up in Rochester, New York. He attended the College and Medical School at the University of Chicago and did residencies in pediatrics, general psychiatry, and child psychiatry and then completed psychoanalytic training. He has received awards from National Institutes of Mental Health (Adolescence and Infancy). He is Retired Freud Professor, The Hebrew University.

War Trauma

Lessons from Israel

Nathan Moses Szajnberg

Routledge
Taylor & Francis Group

LONDON AND NEW YORK

Designed cover image: © Anselm Kiefer, Entfaltung der Sefiroth Unfolding of the Sephirot 1985–1988, 340 x 690 cm 133 7/8 x 271 5/8 in, Oil, acrylic, emulsion, earth, ash, lead, cardboard, metal and fragments of photographs on canvas

First published 2026
by Routledge
4 Park Square, Milton Park, Abingdon, Oxon OX14 4RN

and by Routledge
605 Third Avenue, New York, NY 10158

Routledge is an imprint of the Taylor & Francis Group, an informa business

British Library Cataloguing-in-Publication Data
A catalogue record for this book is available from the British Library

ISBN: 978-1-041-02315-9 (hbk)
ISBN: 978-1-041-01722-6 (pbk)
ISBN: 978-1-003-61869-0 (ebk)

DOI: 10.4324/9781003618690

Typeset in Optima LT Std
by Apex CoVantage, LLC

Dedicated to my wife, Yikun, and four children, Natti, Yadid, Uri, Magnolia Ester, and soon-to-be fifth, Ro'i who tolerated my absence from home while I was in the Negev. My love to my two eldest, Sonia Aviva and Lily Rachel. To my family murdered in the Shoah: all my books are my attempts to give you voices. And to the Jewish people and nation who are also my family.

Contents

Acknowledgments

I am grateful to Professor Gal Meiri, my guide in summer 2024 through the Hellish aftermath of the people of the Negev and to the many generous citizens (including the children of Kibbutz E.) who spoke so openly with me.

I thank Don Beck, photographer extraordinaire, who photographed the children's drawings to capture their clarity.

Kiefer Acknowledgment

We thank Anselm Kiefer, SFMOMA (and donors Doris and Donald Fisher), and the Gagosian Gallery for the "Unfolding of the Sefirot" on the cover.

The unfolding of the Sefirot refers to the Kabbalistic concept of how God's chaotic and void (*Tohu v'vohu*) emanations manifest and interact to create the universe and sustain its existence. Here is a brief overview:

> The Sefirot are ten divine emanations through which the *Ein Sof* (God's Infinite) reveals Himself and continuously creates both the physical and spiritual realms. They are often visualized as a diagram known as the Tree of Life.
>
> In Kabbalah, humans are seen as microcosms of the divine structure; the *sefirot* mirror human qualities, emotions, and actions. Spiritual growth involves aligning one's life with divine attributes.

Kiefer's work has a dark chaos to it, reminding us of how before God created the world, there was void and darkness.

My book focuses on how Israel must unfold its Sefirot from the chaos and darkness of October 7 to recreate its fundamental, millennia-old inherent humanity.

Introduction

What's Personal

"This is personal, this book. After October Seven, I must travel to Israel, be with Jews. **Kol Yisrael Arevim, zeh b'zeh.**" "All Israel is one for the other."

How personal? My father was in the Lodz ghetto, then the Warsaw ghetto until it fell. "Fell," no, destroyed by the Nazis. Then, my father slalomed, like some Swiss speed-skier, through various concentration camps, watching others slain along the slope to Hell, until he reached the ultimate base camp, Auschwitz. Base it was. In the Mengele selection line, my father, barely five foot two, had wrapped toilet paper around his bloody head wound. Mengele with his rider's crop or perhaps only his gloved hands waved my father to the extinction line. My father had noticed who was sent there: the old, the children, the infirm. Quickly, my father ripped off the bloodied head wrap and plunged into the crowd of the labor camp designates. He lasted (as Bellow's Sammler said, "lasted," not "survived") until the Nazis' death marched them out of Auschwitz, the Nazis' attempt to hide their horrors. On this death march, my father, now some 72 pounds, collapsed. Perhaps because the Nazis were in such a rush, they did not shoot him in the head, the usual thing. Some unknown, unknowable soldier—I imagine him as an American—seeing my father still alive, carried him—all 72 pounds—to a Catholic hospital where the nurses still wore wimples, starched white cornettes. Upon awakening and seeing the flying nuns, my father thought he had died and was in heaven.

Because of some quick-eyed, warm-hearted soldier, I am here, writing to you. Born in an American Displaced Persons' Camp in Heidenheim, emigrating to the US sponsored by the Jewish community, educated at the University of Chicago College and Medical School, thanks to the generosity of unknown benefactors, I am here. *Hineini*, "Here I am," as Joseph said to his father when called to find his brothers. *"Hineini,"* as Joseph past Shechem to seek his brothers. I am ready to serve the needs of my Jewish brothers and sisters, and here, to serve you, the reader.

Join me. I ask you to think about the October 7th Hell on Earth, a tour through hell that last some few hours, some too many hours, some 1,200 dead, and others kidnapped by evil. Reflect on how this tour through Hell

DOI: 10.4324/9781003618690-1

has affected not only those who survived (others who only "lasted," we see) but also those Jews in Israel who realize the true evil expressed by Jew-Haters are not only words but actions, and the echoing of Jew-hatred around Europe and the US in particular. (The Far East seems immune thus far to the Jew-hate virus.)[1]

First, let us *see* what may not be unseen. Let us *hear* what has happened, is happening. Western literature recounts other hellish journeys: we will, in this book, recount Odysseus', Aeneus', and Dante's infernal voyages. Then, as with Odysseus', Aeneus', and Dante's journeys through Hell, we will ask what can we learn from horrors.

And, what is our home port? For Odysseus, it was his return to his wife's arms, his son's embrace, and his tree-carved marriage bed. For Aeneus, it cannot be a return; for his home, his Troy is destroyed. He learns in his Hell journey, from his father, that he must find and build a new home in order that his descendants become the greatness of Rome. For Dante, his yearnings are perhaps more modest: to find refuge not only in the arms of his beloved, Heaven-dwelling Beatrice, but also bathed in the light of Christ. We cannot return to October 6; we must build a new psychic home in Israel.

After October 7, where will we find refuge? What will be our home port? Who will accompany us, guide us? Who will embrace us? And in terms of getting through Hell, how do we achieve this voyage? Can we find a guide, preferably a Virgil not some screeching Sybil, to accompany us?

Listen to John Spencer, a soldier/professor of urban warfare[2] on viewing the 45-minute documentation of the Hamas slaughter.

He starts with an experience-distant military description:

"What was done on October 7th was a division level attack[3] . . . division level invasion of Israel by a terrorist Army."

But he descends into more personal reactions:

I have seen my share of evil firsthand around the world in wars of the Middle East, Ukraine, and other areas. I have seen heinous cruelty, dehumanization, and mutilations. I have looked evil men in the eye. *But I have never seen so many evil men (thousands) show such joy in committing their acts.* (My italics)

Thousands of armed marauders gleefully screamed *"Allahu Akhbar!"* as they slashed and burned and tortured and murdered and raped[4] civilians from infants to elderly.

Spencer, a warrior, an officer, was done-in emotionally by watching the 45-minute October 7 documentation, much of it from Moslem GoPros. He—a soldier, a commander—had never seen anything like it. What he had seen was how a unit of his American soldiers would be scarred by the accidental death of a single infant.

What he saw was beyond obscene. Can we find the words to say it? Adorno insisted, *"Nach Auschwitz ein Gedicht zu schreiben, ist barbarisch"* "After Auschwitz, poetry writing is barbaric" (Adorno, 1949/1977). We once thought that writers like Paul Ancel (Celan before the War and his parents' murders flipped his name, and even his identity), Elie Wiesel, and Primo Levi redeemed writing, even poetry after Auschwitz. But after October 7, are there words to say it? And can these words awaken us from that nightmare (and promised future nightmares) to move ourselves into a future free of—free of—what are the words for it? Free of what?! What?! If October 7 (and its after-shocks) *were* a nightmare, we would awaken with all those murdered and kidnapped alive. If it were a nightmare, we could sort it out and move into a safer future for ourselves and our children. But the words of Hamas/Iran/Hezbollah and its American/European apologist proxies (AOC/Tlaib/Ilhan, etc.) promise us that they will make these nightmarish *acts* recur. We can never return to whom we were on October 6. In any case, those slaughtered remain dead.

These are some of the questions I ask us to consider in this book. Prior to October 7, I was writing a book on expression of emotions in Western Art over two millennia, an exploration of the history of emotions that Darwin argued were evolutionary and that Ekman and colleagues showed were universal. I dropped that on October 8th. I began an exploration of the hellish journeys of our Western traditions—Odysseus, Aeneus, and Danté in order to learn from them. That is the first chapter of this book. Chapter 2 is how can we use wisdom literature and our experiences to overcome the living nightmare of October 7 (and promise of further annihilations) to build a better future. In December 2023 and after, in the summer of 2024, I spent time in the Negev, along the Gaza border and among the evacuated children and families, consulting with IDF soldiers. I describe the evacuated children and show their drawings and stories in Chapter 3. Chapter 4 is on treating soldiers in the denseness of war. My IDF colleagues describe how to "build" a clinic for traumata in a war zone, and how to treat acute traumatic disorder of war under falling bombs. The last chapter describes the returning *Otef* (Gaza border) communities and how to rebuild the parents and their communities, even as they still yearn and mourn for the slaughtered and for the kidnapped, even as they repair bullet holes and shrapnel-shattered windows and rebuild their children's shelters.

Join me on this journey.

These are the questions I seek to address with you, the reader. To learn what we can from Odysseus, Aeneus, and Danté—also from the children, the parents, the soldiers (who are fathers and sons, daughters and mothers) about how to emerge from Hell, about the future, and about a safe haven.

This book feels rushed. When I wrote my soldier book (2006), I was almost done when the Lebanese Two war broke out. I decided I couldn't finish the book until I'd spoken with my soldiers about being called to fight in Lebanon (along with most of my University students).

But this war, this conflagration? When will it be done? This has become the longest war in Israeli's modern history. Over 800 soldiers are dead as of this writing, let alone the thousands of Israeli civilians including some dozen Druze soccer-playing children in one fell swoop. I cannot wait to write until it is over. Hopefully, by the time you read this book, we will be in the aftermath. Then we enter a new phase, not only treating those in war, but after war, perhaps an "easier," but not easy task. To rebuild a nation. Let us learn from those who suffer and think about how to repair the soul of a nation.

Notes

1 China's anti-Israel stance seems to be a Communist Party phenomenon, not one of the populace.
2 John Spencer is chair of urban warfare studies at the Modern War Institute (MWI) at West Point, codirector of MWI's Urban Warfare Project, and host of the "Urban Warfare Project Podcast." He served for 25 years as an infantry soldier, which included two combat tours in Iraq. He is the author of the book "Connected Soldiers: Life, Leadership, and Social Connection in Modern War" and co-author of "Understanding Urban Warfare."
3 Some 4,000 armed men, trained to attack civilians. Trained to evoke terror.
4 Can the word "rape" capture what was done to these women: their pelvises pulverized, their legs ripped from their sockets, their blood-soaked clothes screaming, "There must be a different word." See Sheryl Sandberg's "Silent Screams" (2024).

1   Wisdom From Ancient Texts on Hellish Journeys?

How can we emerge from the Hell on Earth of October 7? More specifically, as a developmental psychiatrist, I ask, how do we rebuild our children's lives to emerge from their hells?

To begin to answer this, I reach back several millennia, into wisdom literature, to remember three hellish journeys of Antique times: Odysseus, Aeneas, and Danté. Each was told to go through Hell to learn how to live better lives, how to build futures. Jews don't shy away from learning from wisdom literature even if millennia old. Let us begin our journeys then, there.

Midway through life's journey, Odysseus's hellish attempt to return home, in book 11 of 24, Odysseus descends to the Underworld. His seven-year lover, Calypso, had predicted this interlude. Recall that *The Odyssey*, despite its name, does not introduce Odysseus until the fifth book. The first four books detail the real, societal decay of Ithacan society since King Odysseus's reluctant departure with Menelaus and Agamemnon to retrieve the "kidnapped" Helen from Troy and Paris's amorous arms. We cannot review the entire epic here but offer an overview to begin to understand the necessity for Odysseus' exploration of Hell.

Not until Book Five do we meet Odysseus. He proceeds in the next four to five books through a series of fantastical, even supernatural adventures (let us say, even dreamlike). He dwells with his lover Calypso for seven years, which he experiences as seven days; she, a demi-human who promises him eternal life if only he would remain (and possibly love her). Then, he shipwrecks naked on the Island of the Phaecians, a group of demi-humans who consort with the gods, who are the creation of Poseidon (an avowed enemy of Odysseus's return) and live a fantasy-like almost Edenic life. There, beginning in Book Nine, Odysseus flexes not only his rhetorical muscle, at their insistence, narrating his adventures including his Troy battle, but also his blinding of the Cyclops (another of Poseidon's offspring) and struggle against the lotus-eaters, whose fruit induces forgetting, his struggle against the Sirens, and his ship-wrenching struggle between Scylla and Charybdis. Odysseus is a tale-spinner, an entrancer.

The lotus-eaters episode reminds us that memory serves three contending vectors in *The Odyssey*: (1) memory magnetizes Odysseus homeward;

DOI: 10.4324/9781003618690-2

(2) memory haunts and jeopardizes the present if the "past" is experienced *as* present;[1] or (3) memory is aborted and halts this journey, forgetting the past (by eating the lotus).

After the series of fantastical adventures, some described by Homer, some rhapsodized by Odysseus at the Phaecians' request, Odysseus begins his truer return home when washed naked, a true "nobody," on Ithaca's shores. By Book Twelve, we enter the world of reality.

But Book Eleven, our focus here contains Odysseus' sojourn he must make through the Underworld. This is prophesied, even encouraged, by Calypso and Circe, in order to consult with Tiresias, that blind, once man/once woman/again man, seer who will help navigate Odysseus's final travel. Let's look at this necessary descent into the underworld to better understand what Odysseus learns here, whom he meets, and how it furthers his ardent desire to return "home." In short, how does this dreamlike underworld descent better prepare, even awaken Odysseus to return to his desired reality?

Circe advises Odysseus to take the Underworld detour: how to enter it with blood spilled on the ground, how to avoid the onslaught of a myriad of ghosts eager to engage him, and to listen well to Tiresias, "whose reason is still unshaken" (Book X). Circe is the counterpart to Calypso, but Odysseus has matured since Calypso. With Calypso, Odysseus is seduced to stay for seven years, although he spends much of the time weeping at the beach for his Ithaca/Penelope. As Odysseus refuses eternal life, Calypso promises Odysseus that she will release him of her own will; a confabulation, as she has been visited by Hermes and commanded to release him. Even after agreeing to his departure, she does not actively help, rather simply permits him to gather wood for his watercraft. Like Noah, he builds his own ark, but filled with his men, every one of whom will soon perish under his command (although he demurs, only because they disobeyed his orders).

Circe entices Odysseus for but a year. From the beginning, he is "on to" her transformational tricks, her toxic potion that has turned his men into pigs, impulsive filthy animals. He resists her, that is, but does bed her when she reassures him, she will not "unman" him in bed. And Circe releases Odysseus of her own will, even aiding him with supplies including a ram and black ewe for Tiresias's sacrifice, and more importantly, sage advice. She blows a steady wind "dead aft" to guide him to Hell.

We suggest reading the Underworld journey like a nightmare/dream. (But we also suggest that we can read much of Odysseus' ten-year return as a nightmare/dream following the real-life nightmarish *Iliad* exploits over ten years warring against Troy.)[2]

At the permanently dusk mistiness of Hell's gate, "where the sun never pierces," Odysseus makes proper offerings, finally pouring the blood of the ewe run into a trench dug by him. Spilled blood pivots us—Janus-faced, it points us to the past *Iliad*, when Odysseus (and cohort) spilled blood (at Helena's "feet"), and it points us to the future suitors' blood that he will spill in his courtyard at his wife, Penelope's "feet." But here, now, his sword should be drawn, Circe warns him, to protect himself from the onslaught of ghosts. He abides by Circe's advice to speak with each ghost individually.

He is accosted:

the tribes of the dead came up and gathered round me in their tens of thousands, raising their eerie cry. *Their panic* turned me pale, gripped by the sudden fear that *dread Persephone might send me up from* Hades' Halls some ghastly monster like the Gorgon's head (My emphasis).
(Book XI; Homer, Odyssey, Fagles, 1990)

He recalls Circe's advice to speak to each individually.

And he does. Elpenor speaks, the unfortunate young soldier, who awakening from a drunken stupor, fell, broke his neck, and descended to Hell without a proper burial.

Then quaffing the blood, Tiresias prophesies. Odysseus's return home will not be soon and only "if you can restrain yourself and your companions, at the cattle-filled Island of the sun god" (Book XI; Homer, Odyssey, Fagles, 1990). Odysseus must restrain his hunger and his famished soldiers in order to reach homeward. This tension between oral gorging and restraint is a recurrent theme in the Odyssey: at feasts, husbands are cuckolded (Helen's "abduction" by Paris) or 108 suitors slaughtered by Odysseus (after they have repeatedly transgressed the concept of "Xenia");[3] his soldiers gluttonously gobble-up Circe's magic potions and become pigs; and ultimately defy Odysseus, yielding to their stomachs by eating the 350 eternally living cattle of the God; even at the 108 suitors final feast, Odysseus shoots arrows through their gullets.[4] Tiresias continues: if his men harm this flock, both they and Odysseus's ship will be destroyed, and Odysseus will return, but "in bad plight." Tiresias informs Odysseus of the disorder at his home, "overrun by high-handed people . . . devouring your substance . . . making presents to your wife." In a part prophesy, part command, Tiresias continues, "you will take your revenge on these suitors." But even then, Odysseus's journey will not be complete, not after killing the suitors, not after meeting his son, not after reuniting with his wife, and not even after seeing his aged father. Odysseus must bear an oar and come to a country of people, "who have never heard of the sea . . . do not mix salt with their food, . . . know anything about ships, nor oars, . . . the wings of a ship" (Book XI; Homer, Odyssey, Fagles, 1990). The latter is a tall order for a Greek, a nation known for its seafarers. He is later released by the gods from this command/curse.

Then, in a moment of softening warmth, Odysseus' mother appears. Downcast, she seems not to recognize him. Odysseus implores Tiresias: how can he get his mother to speak? And Tiresias reminds him, to hear his now-silent mother's ghost to recognize and speak to him, she must drink his blood offering.

Listen to one of the more poignant moments in Hades.

His mother begins with questions: why is her son among the dead? Has he not seen his wife or his home?

After brief answers, Odysseus asks her of *her* death "tell me, tell me true." He asks about his father, his wife, his son, and his estate.

The mother starts with the living; his wife is in tears day and night, his estate intact, his son alive, and his father isolated far from town, sleeping on the floor in rags or in the vineyards in the summer. "He grieves continually about your never having come home."

And of her death? Here are her words only in part:

> my longing to know what you were doing and the force of my affection for you—this was the death of me.
>
> (Book XI; Homer, Odyssey, Fagles, 1990)

She died of heartbreak, missing Odysseus.

We sense a pang of superego guilt.

His response touches our hearts and reminds us of how this is dreamlike.

> I tried to find some way of embracing my poor mother's ghost. Thrice I sprang towards her and tried to clasp her in my arms, but each time she flitted from my embrace as if it were a *dream or phantom*.' Mother, why do you not stay still when I would embrace you? If we could throw our arms around one another, we might find sad comfort in the sharing of our sorrows even in the house of Hades; does Proserpine want to lay a still further load of grief upon me by mocking me with a phantom only? (Au. Italics).

Odysseus tells us this seems like and feels like a dream. We are launched by his words to understand that much of this is dreamlike. Odysseus emerges from the surrealistic years with fantastical women, Calypso and Circe, to the more subjectively dreamlike encounter with the other woman in his past life, his mother. Perhaps we are being prepared in this "dream" for his ultimate reunion with that second woman in his life, Penelope.

His mother's sage response? "The soul flits as though it were a dream." And she adds, as she launches his barque, "note all these things that you may tell them to your wife hereafter." That is, we might speculate: gather up the dreamlike knowledge to apply to your lived, awake life with wisdom. This hero's barque is launched to Hell by one woman but launched homeward by another, his mother.

All the previous trip to the underworld is narrated by Odysseus to entertain his hosts: we are interrupted by Alcinous, king of the Phaecians and Odysseus' host, who demands more of the tale. Whereupon Odysseus continues this oneiric account by dismissing the female ghosts to have Agamemnon enter the stage. His tale of murder so foul is repeated thrice in the Odyssey. And a wife is central to his tale, is the start of the Trojan War with Helena's abduction: Achilles' pouting at the start of the Iliad when his slave girl is abducted by Agamemnon (brother of the cuckolded Menelaus) after Achilles rightly insists that Agamemnon return a daughter as demanded by the gods.

Agamemnon gets is rightly due upon being both cuckolded and then killed by his wife and her lover. Agamemnon never connects his being cuckolded with his brother's own theft of a woman and his murderous threats to Achilles. This synthetic work is left to the reader/listener.[5]

After detailing the gore of his death, "mixing bowl (of wine) and the loaded tables . . . the gourd reeking with our blood," Agamemnon closes with bitter advice (like some later Polonius)

> be not be too friendly even with your own wife . . . Tell her a part only and your own counsel about the rest . . . do not tell people when you are bringing your ship to Ithaca, but steal a march upon them . . . there is no trusting women.

Finally, Homer returns us to the start of the Iliad, the rage of Achilles by introducing his ghost whose plaintive closing words speak to the over-glorification of war. When Odysseus tries to glorify Achilles' heroic death, Achilles responds all too wisely:

Say not a word in death's favor. . . . I would rather be a paid servant in a poor man's house and be above ground than king of kings among the dead.

When Achilles then asks about his son, this ghost father reveals his true concerns, as do the ghosts in the third text we read, Danté's *Inferno*, such as the Tuscan entombed, aflame Cavalcanté (5278).

When Achilles hears of his son's heroism and being alive, he "strode off across a meadow full of asphodel, exulting over what I had said concerning the progress of his son." We can at least ask, was it his son's progress or his son's survival that moved Achilles, who would rather be an alive servant than an adulated dead hero?

After Odysseus reconciles with the still-petulant Ajax over Odysseus's victory about the armor of Achilles, after seeing Sisyphus "at his endless task," a task that reminds us of Odysseus's god-rebuffed voyages homeward, he is accosted by "mighty Hercules" who spoke piteously, "My poor Odysseus . . . are you too leading the same sorry kind of life that I did when I was above ground . . . through an infinity of suffering." We can remember Odysseus being named by his grandfather after the word for pain, for until now, we hear much of his pain (if we put aside his eight years of seduction by Calypso and Circe). Only then, does Odysseus realize that he must escape Hades or be overwhelmed by the myriad of mighty dead "thousands of ghosts came round me and uttered such appalling cries that I was panic-stricken." He feared that awful monster Gorgon who might pursue him and Odysseus retreats to his boat, rowing at first (one must labor, back-breaking rowing to escape this nightmarish Hades) until "a fair wind sprang up." Recall this feared Gorgon: the three sisters of Greek mythology, Stheno, Euyale, and better-known Medusa, whose snake hair would turn the living into stone, who would freeze

Odysseus to this place in Hell for eternity. He escapes the nightmarish world to launch himself into the awake world of his external reality.

We but summarize the remaining dozen books of the Odyssey if only to give a flavor of how the underworld, oneiric world changed Odysseus's actions in his return to reality. All his men cannot restrain their hunger on the God's cattle isle, gorge, and are murdered. Odysseus is discovered stark naked and washed ashore, by Nausicaa, daughter of the king. He treats her with remarkable restraint, particularly after his dalliances with Calypso and Circe. She too is modest and restrained and guides him to their castle. Then, after demonstrating his rhetorical shine to the Phaecians, Odysseus is taunted to show his physical progress and outshines them again. But the Phaecians *play* games; Odysseus *is* a warrior.

This restraint is a foretaste of what he will show when he arrives on the beaches of Ithaca; veiled by Athena's induced mist and fog, he doesn't know where he is; doesn't recognize his homeland. Like someone awakening from deep dreams, he blunders (but with Athena by him) until he meets his devoted pig herder, Eumaeus. From Circe's pigs to those owned by his estate but guarded by loyal Eumaeus, Odysseus gradually awakens, first to meet his son, then, disguised, to visit his estate, to assess the 108 suitors and plan out their demise, to meet his Penelope, who appears not to recognize him, and to shoot his arrow through the axe holes, before he immediately sets out to slaughter all the suitors and even hang those maidservants, their legs kicking like throttled doves, who had bedded down the suitors. We have an abrupt ending echoing the *Iliad*, of war and the man.

Our Next Hellish Sojourn: *The Aeneid*

Let us turn to the *Aeneid*, which we will consider an offspring of *The Iliad* and *Odyssey*. For, not only did Aeneas survive the destruction of his Troy and found the Roman civilization but also the poet, Virgil, was moved by Homer to continue the tale. There are parallels and significant differences between the two, which we will but note here. We will dwell on Aeneas's sojourn through the Underworld and also found midway through his journey recounted in the epic poem.

Aeneas is often called *pietas*, which has a wider meaning in Latin such as "dutiful" mindful of one's duty "to the gods, one's family and to one's country." Let's recall that Odysseus, in contrast, is *polytropos*, of many shapes, wiley, a deceiver. We have already a distinction in character between the two heroes. To skip to the end, Aeneas arrives at the future home of Rome with his men intact, as opposed to Odysseus, *all* of whose men die in his charge, who arrives alone and naked, a "nobody."

We begin with Troy crumbling about him. Aeneas thinks to leave, but his father, Anchises refuses. When Aeneas says he'll stay to fight, his wife Creusa reminds him of the fate of their son, Ancises. The boy suddenly is aflame and Aeneas, taking this as an omen from the gods, chooses to escape. With his father astride Aeneas's shoulders, his son by the hand, and Creusa following, they leave. She quickly falls behind and is killed. Aeneas returns to find her but finds her ghost which prophesies that Aeneas will get another wife. Thrice Aeneas tries to embrace her, only to find ghostly mist. In this brief introduction to Aeneas, we have a rapid sketch of his *pietas*, his dutiful character.

In the first five books, prior to his descent, Aeneas meets Dido, who falls deeply in love with him, and Aeneas can show his rhetorical chops, akin to Odysseus, as he recites the fall of Troy and his journey. Dido famously kills herself when Aeneas chooses to leave. When, later, Aeneas meets her shade in the underworld, he bawls tearfully for her forgiveness. Intriguingly such a heartfelt crying is absent at Creusa's death. Dido's shade slumps away wordlessly, angrily.

In book five, Aeneas holds funeral games for the first anniversary of his father's death. Only after this can he enter his underworld journey.[6]

Aeneas is "facilitated" by his guide, the Cumaean Sibyl, a priestess and prophetess; she accompanies, at times guides, him in Hell. But she is no benign *Baedeker*. As Aeneas approaches with Apollo at his side, listen to the Sibyl's reaction:

Suddenly, all her features, all her color changes, her braided hair flies loose and her breast heaves, her heart bursts with frenzy . . . the ring of her voice no longer human, the breath the power of god comes closer, closer. "Why so slow Trojan Aeneas?' She shouts, 'so slow to pray to swear your vows?"

(Virgil, VI, 65 ff Barsch 2021)

And the hero's response?

An icy shiver runs through the Trojan's sturdy spines and the king's prayers come pouring from his heart: 'Apollo, you always pitied the Trojans' heavy labors! You guided the arrow of Paris, and pierced Achilles' body. You led me through many seas, bordering endless coasts . . . Let the doom of Troy pursue us just this far, no more . . . you blessed Sibyl who knows the future, grant my prayer. I ask no more than the realm my fate decrees: let the Trojans rest in Latium, . . . And Sibyl for you too a magnificent sacred shrine awaits you in our kingdom. . . . Just don't commit your words to the rustling, scattering leaves—sport of the winds that whirl them all away. Sing them yourself, I beg you!

(Virgil, VI, 65 ff Barsch 2021)

But the Sibyl, remaining unbent,

storms with a wild fury . . . the more she tries to pitch the great god off her breast, the more his bridle exhausts her raving lips, overwhelming her untamed heart, bending her to his will.

(Virgil VI, 93 ff Barsch 2021)

Whereupon, she prophesies;

> you Trojans will reach Laviniums' realm—but you will rue your arrival. Wars, horrendous wars, and the Tiber foaming with tides of blood, I see it all!. . . and the cause of this, this new Trojan grief? Again a stranger bride, a marriage with a stranger once again.
>
> (Virgil VI, 102 ff; Barsch 2021)

Aeneas boldly claims that he will withstand all this future strife, and then poignantly asks of her, "allow me to go and see my beloved father . . . teach me the way throw wide the sacred doors." He continues:

> Through fires, a thousand menacing spears I swept him off on these shoulders and saved him from our enemies' onslaught. He shared all roads and he braved all seas with me, all threats of the waves and skies . . . graced with a strength beyond his years . . . he was the one . . . who ordered, pressed me on to reach your doors and seek you, beg you now. Pity the son and father, I pray you, kindly lady! All power is yours . . . If Orpheus could summon up the ghost of his wife . . . if Pollux could ransom his brother . . . If Theseus, mighty Hercules . . . I too can trace my birth from Jove on high. So he prayed, grasping the altar.
>
> (Virgil VI 125 ff; Barsch 2021)

Sibyl answers with words we will remember and even apply to the descent into the underworld of nightmarish dreams and our attempt to ascend from them with meaning.

> The descent to the Underworld is easy. Night and day the gates of the shadowy Death stand open wide. *But to retrace your steps, to climb back to the upper air—there the struggle, there the labor lies.* Only a few, loved by impartial Jove or borne aloft to the sky *by their own fiery virtue*—some sons of the gods have made their way. The entire heartland here is thick with woods. Cocytus glides around it coiling dense and dark. But if such a wild desire seizes on you—twice to sail the Stygian marsh, to see black Tartarus twice—If you're so eager to give yourself to this, *this mad ordeal*, then hear what you must accomplish first (My emphasis).
>
> (Virgil VI, 149 ff; Barsch 2021)

Death, the Sibyl warns, is easy and available to all mortals; *returning to life* after (psychic death, for living Aeneas) is the struggle; "there the labor lies," available to those with fiery virtue. What labor, what struggles, we have only begun to taste and we will learn with time.

The Sibyl stipulates his first acts. Pick the Golden Bough to offer to Proserpina; second, bury a friend who "lies dead—oh you would not know—his body pollutes your entire fleet" (Virgil VI, 149 ff; Barsch 2021). The Sibyl cautions silver-tongued Aeneas that his rhetorical virtues are not sufficient; he must perform acts to even enter Hades.

Aeneas has different escorts as his darker journey begins. His trusted comrade Achates and he ponder over who might have died. The Sibyl shows us that while she can lead Aeneas, he will need to work, to discover what he needs to move into and through Hell. When they "discover" Misenus' body, Aeneas orders the elaborate funeral rites. Then, two doves are beseeched by Aeneas to help find the Golden Bough beyond the "foul-smelling gorge" (Virgil VI, 149 ff; Barsch 2021).

But Aeneas' consistent guide is the now-transformed Sibyl. At her commands, he "slaughters a black-fleeced lamb to the Furies' mother, Night, and her great sister, Earth and to you, Proserpina, kills a barren heifer." Others are slaughtered for other gods. Only then, does the Sibyl proclaim, "Now for courage, now the steady heart!" And plunges into the yawning cave of Hell. Aeneas "follows her boldly, matching stride for stride, proclaiming: 'You gods who govern the realm of ghosts . . . reveal the world immersed in the misty depths of earth'" (Virgil VI, 149 ff; Barsch 2021). Words we might use today to demand that our oneiric world be revealed.

Immediately at the entryway,

> Grief and the pangs of Conscience make their beds, and fatal pale Disease lives there and bleak Old Age, Dread and Hunger, seductress to crime and grinding Poverty . . . and Death and deadly struggle, and Sleep, twin brother of Death and twisted wicked Joys and facing them at the threshold, War, rife with death and the Furies' iron chambers and mad raging Strife, whose blood-stained headbands knot her snaky locks.
> (Virgil VI, 149 ff; Barsch 2021)

The modern reader notes that these capitalized pains of life are not abstract nouns—rather, Grief, Conscience, Disease and Hunger, Old Age, grinding Poverty, Death, and "Sleep, the brother of Death"—were experienced as tormenting gods, attacks coming from the outside world (although experienced as internal suffering).

Aeneas is accosted by "swarms of false dreams" as well as half-beasts, and half-monsters—Centaurs, Scylla, Chimera, and Gorgons and Harpies. One task, we gather, is that Aeneas must dissect false from true dreams, as we will see nearing the end of his Hell journey.

Aeneas' initial impulse is to grip his sword, not realizing at the moment that these are "disembodied creatures . . . empty phantoms."

Only now does Aeneas reach Charon and the dreaded crossing in his "red-rust skiff" the River Styx to Hell proper.

On his shore, Aeneas sees throngs of ghosts begging to be borne by Charon across and refused by him. Sibyl explains that these are the unburied who will remain here for eternity or until their bones are interred (today, we might speculate until they are mourned properly). He spies his pilot Palinurus, swept off in the night, tiller in hand into the ocean, washed ashore in Italy, and then murdered by brigands. Palinurus shows his character when he says that when driven overboard, he feared less for himself than for his shipmates now in a tiller-less ship.

At critical moments, the Sibyl aids Aeneas. Charon spies the living Aeneas and demands, "Stop . . . Why have you come? Speak up . . . not one step more! This is the realm of shadows, sleep, and drowsy night" (Virgil VI, 200 ff; Barsch 2021).

Whereupon, Sibyl, Apollo's seer, chimes

> There's not treachery here—just calm down . . . (this is) Aeneas of Troy famous for his devotion, feats of arms goes down to the deepest shades of hell to see his father." And, sensing that her rhetoric is not persuasive, she offers the Golden Bough, "the ferryman, marveling at the awesome gift.

As we progress into Aeneas' Hell, we learn that it is highly differentiated compared to Odysseus'. First, we have seen the multiple gateways prior to crossing the River Styx—caves of thousands of mouths;[7] half-beasts, the human afflictions of Grief, Conscience, Disease, Old Age; and unburied ghosts crowding the shore.

Now we progress at first through ghosts of infants weeping, "snatched from the breast on that black day," or those condemned to die on false charges; next, sad ghosts, innocents all who brought death by their own hands, now yearning for the world above. Then, Sibyl points out the Fields of Mourning: souls consumed by wasting sickness, and cruel love, such as Caeneus, even a once young man, now a woman. (We recall Tiresias of *The Odyssey* who reappears to Aeneas.) And finally, Aeneas sees Dido, "wound still fresh."

We hear Aeneas mourn as we have not heard him following his wife's or his father's deaths.

> Tragic Dido,. . . you took final measure with a sword . . . was it I who caused your death? I swear by the stars . . . (that) I left your shores my Queen against my will. Yes, there will of the gods . . . Stay a moment. Don't withdraw from my sight . . . Aeneas . . . with welling tears tried to soothe her rage.
>
> (Virgil VI, 540 ff)

The reader/listener hears that *this* Aeneas is not yet prepared to take more responsibility for leaving Dido and leading her to suicide; Aeneas is still at the beginning of his Hell journey of (self) discovery.

"But she, her eyes fixed on the ground turned away, her features no more moved by his pleas . . . as if she were set in stony flint or Parian marble . . . his enemy forever" (Virgil VI 545 ff).

The Underworld shifts beneath our feet as "labor(ing) along the charted path . . . They gain the utmost lower fields where throngs of the great war heroes live apart." We hear a differentiation from a hellish setting to the Elysian, a paradisal place for heroes. We soon will enter a realm more familiar to Aeneas.

But note, before we leave the segmented levels of Aeneas's Hell, that when we turn to Danté later, Danté builds upon Virgil's infrastructure and even differentiates the levels of hell further, sin by sin.

In the heroes' circle, of the many met, Aeneas dwells on mutilated Deiphobus, Priam's son. We see his disfiguration: face hacked to pieces, ears ripped off, and nostrils slashed "He can hardly recognize him." And as Aeneas hears Deiphobus's account of the "deadly crimes of that Spartan whore (Helena)" Aeneas weeps.

As Dawn reaches her zenith and Night approaches—Time passes for Aeneas in this timeless Underworld—Sibyl reprimands the weeping Aeneas.

> We waste our time with tears. This is the place where the road divides in two. To the right it runs below the mighty walls of Death, our path to Elysium, to the left hand road torment the wicked leading down to Tartarus, path to doom.
>
> (Virgil VI, 609 ff Barsch 2021)

The Sibyl, like Athena with sobbing Odysseus and Telemachus on each other's shoulders, has only so much patience for weeping. Move on to action.

Emitting from Tartarus' River of Fire, Aeneas hears groans, "the savage crack of the lash, grating creak of iron, clank of dragging chains." He freezes (VI 645 ff Barsch 2021).

"Tell me Sibyl, what are the punishments . . .?"

"Famous captain of Troy, no pure soul may set foot on that wicked threshold . . . the Cretan Rhadamanthus rules with an iron hand, censuring men, exposing fraud, forcing confessions . . . of hidden crimes." Finally, these souls are faced with the monstrous Hydra, "fifty black maws gaping" before being plunged into the Tartarus abyss. There the Titan's spawn

> writhe in the deep pit . . . Tityus too . . . that son of Earth . . . his giant body splayed out over nine whole acres, a hideous vulture . . . gorging down his immortal liver and innards . . . Deep in his chest, it nestles, ripping into its feast and the fibers grown afresh, gets no relief from pain. . . . Here are those who hated their brothers . . . or struck their fathers . . . or embroiled clients in fraud . . . killed for adultery . . . marched to the flag of civil war.

"Don't hunger, to know their doom" she cautions. Yet she tells him of their doom: "trundling enormous boulders, others dangle, racked to the breaking point on the spokes of rolling wheels." She ends by adding to the sins, "one

who forced himself on his daughter's bed and sealed a forbidden marriage."[8]
"Not if I had a hundred tongues and a hundred mouths and a voice of iron . . .
I could never capture all the crimes or run through all the torments doom by
doom" (Virgil Vi, 720–27; Barsch 2021).

Now, Aeneas rinses his limbs with pure water and plants the Golden
Bough. They transition to the "Fortunate Groves where the blessed make their
homes" (VI, 742). He prepares to seek his father, Anchises. He scans the past
heroes, Orpheus with his seven-string lyre, poets "whose songs were fit for
Phoebus,"[9] others flexing their limbs in wrestling rings or grappling on golden
sands, dance, and chant.

Father Anchises? He's found reviewing souls "eagerly *on the way* to the
world of light above . . . his own people, all his cherished heirs" (Virgil VI,
785 ff; Barsch 2021).

We will soon learn from Anchises what he must teach Aeneas about his
future efforts, and his upcoming travails.

But first, we have a poignant moment: Anchises glimpses his son.

> he reached out both his hands as his spirit lifted, tears ran down his
> cheeks, a cry broke for his lips: "You've come at last? Has the love your
> father hoped for mastered the hardship of the journey? Let me look at
> your face, my son."

Unlike Odysseus's mother who almost looks through him at first, voiceless,
until she can slake her blood thirst, Anchises is enlivened by seeing his son.
Aeneas explains,

> "Your grieving ghost so often it came and urged me to your threshold."
> So Aeneas pleaded his face streaming tears. Three times he tried to fling
> his arms around his neck, three times he embraced—nothing, a phan-
> tom sifting through his fingers lights as wind, *quick as a dream* in flight.
> (Virgil, VI, 800–10; My emphasis; Barsch 2021)

Listen to the poet and think of all this, all this journey, is, as Odysseus too
said, a dream or dreamlike.

Now, Aeneas sees that they are by the River Lethe, the stream of forgetfulness, and asks his father about this and this throng of souls "like bees in
meadowlands" (VI, 815; Barsch 2021) hovering by.

Father gives two answers, one general that reveals the possibility of rein-
carnation, the other specific, about the heirs of Anchises should Aeneas complete his journey and responsibilities.

"They are the spirits owed a second body by the Fates. They drink deep
of the River of Lethe . . . that will set them . . . oblivious forever" (Virgil, VI,
825ff Barsch 2021). But prior to this quaff of forgetfulness that prepares them
for return to earthly life, the souls must undergo rigorous purification of "their
stains, their crimes" sorted away by fire, or splayed out before empty winds
or planned in rushing floods. As with *The Odyssey*, memory or its loss is

important. For Virgil's Hell, memory loss is necessary for rebirth, but not for Aeneus. He, we will see, must remember well in order to know his future.

"Each of us must suffer his own demanding ghost," Anchises states, including himself among the stained (Virgil, VI, 859; Barsch 2021). Even then this process takes a thousand years.

Aeneas asks why anyone would want to return to "the shackles of the body," this "mad desire . . . for the light of life?"

We can speculate here whether Aeneas is tempted to remain with his father, united in these Elysian Fields, rather than return earthward and to his upcoming travails "shut up in the body's tomb, a prison dark and deep" (849). As if to persuade Aeneas to pursue his voyage and tasks on earth, Anchises gives this second answer, a litany of the heirs lined up before them, preparing to be inspected by Anchises, future heroes of Rome and Italy, Aeneas's offspring.

We can read the River Lethe passage as an analog to the lotus-eaters—past forgetting. If Aeneas forgets his past, or forgets this underworld, oneiric voyage, he will lose his drive to find a new home. He will stay blissfully stagnant for a millennium, so too if we forgot our dreams, or what we learn from them. But we can demand further, since Aeneas will return to the world above, is he expected to be cleansed of some memories, while retaining others?

"Come," Anchises says,

the glory that will follow the sons of Troy through time, your children born of Italian stock who wait for life, bright souls, future heirs of our name and our renown. I will reveal them all and tell you of your fate.
(Virgil, VI, 878 ff.; Barsch 2021)

And we hear the litany of the future—Cesar, Romulus, Marcellus, and Numa (who established Roman law).

Yet wise Anchises also cautions his Aeneas against civil war, citing Cesar and his son-in-law, Pompey's, battle.

Anchises finishes his recitation, his exhortation to his son:

You, Roman, remember, rule with all your power the peoples of the earth—*these will be your arts*: to put your stamp on the works and ways of peace, to spare the defeated, break the proud in war.
(Virgil, VI, 980 ff.; My emphasis; Barsch 2021)

Now, we learn *why* Anchises was driven to voyage through Hell in order to complete his journey. He needed not only to see his father but also to hear the endpoint, the purpose of his journey: not only to reach a new shore, a new home, but also to establish the empire of Rome and how to rule. The future heirs and greatness will fill Aenea's sails and give him proper direction. He "knows" how to navigate to Hesperia, the gods will guide his navigation, and he "knows" that he will learn where to set permanent anchor based on his living father's prophesy: when his men are so famished that they eat their dishes, Aeneas will know to make permanent camp.[10] But from his father's ghost, he learns the true motivation for his final journey. His father serves as the ego ideal who gives not only hope but a sense of promising future of inspiration, "inspired," almost literally a deep breath of air.

There are twin Gates of Sleep to exit the Underworld, the same two mentioned in *The Odyssey*. Gates of Sleep are called, as if to underline, to emphasize the *dream* experiences we have heard. The first is the Gate of Horn for "true shades," which offers easy passage. The other "glistens with ivory, radiant, flawless, but through it the dead send false dreams up towards the sky" (1032; Barsch 2021). Intriguingly, Anchises escorts his son and Sibyl through the Ivory Gate. This makes sense. Aeneas is not a shade and is not a dream: he is the only living being (Sibyl is a prophetess, demigod) passing through this Underworld. He must pass the Gates of Sleep as a "false dream" (1034; Barsch 2021) sent by the dead—for he is alive and will live. Just as we too pass from the Gates of Sleep into living reality and if we are fortunate, persistent, and successful, *if we have some guidance*, we can make sense of our travel and travails through the shady underworld of Sleep.

Let's take a moment before we leave Aeneas's Sleepwalk through the dream world, to compare Aeneas's experience with his father-ghost to Odysseus with his mother-ghost. For, Virgil builds upon Homer, not mimic him.

Odysseus goes to the Underworld to seek prophesy/advice from that hermaphroditic, blinded seer, Tiresias. By happenstance, Odysseus meets his mother, whom he doesn't know, nor is told, has died. As mentioned earlier, she does not "see" him or speak to him until he offers the blood he has brought. She does not prophesy his future, except to tell him of the present— his estate is intact, his wife alive, and his father in mourning. From this, Odysseus can build an anticipation of some near future. He does not, like Aeneas, "see" generations emerging from his loins or efforts; he only strengthens his resolve to return to his past.[11]

Aeneas begs to see his father. Even though he "knows" he will be navigated to his new shores. Even though he "knows" from his living father's hint how he will recognize these shores. He simply yearns to see him. And upon doing so he learns that some souls desire to return to the "tomb" of their fleshy, earthly selves. To do so, they undergo an excruciating millennium of cleansing—their skins splayed out, scorched, or winds howling through them. Then, he learns from his father the true reason for him to labor through his journey and furthermore, to withstand the future battles of his new homeland. His guide, the screeching, banshee Sibyl, is converted first by Aeneas's emollient words and then by his Golden Bough. Aeneas, unlike Odysseus, must earn his entrance to Hell, must pass through multiple gates before meeting his desired being, his father.

Through Danté's Infernal *Inferno*, Guided by Virgil, *En Route* to the Arms of Beatrice in Paradise

The Inferno was written some 1.5 millennia after Virgil's *Aeneid*, but leans on it and elaborates it. The five letters—D-A-N-T-´E—make writers tremble to compose even an overview of his underworld. Auerbach (1967) pronounced the

Commedia and its *Inferno* as the greatest work of literature. But let us keep in mind both the past—Homer and Virgil—and the future oneiric explorer, Freud.

At first, the reader might object: *The Inferno* is the *first* of the three books of the *Commedia*; unlike the Odyssey (or the Iliad) or Aeneid, it doesn't start *in media res*, in the middle of the journey. And the hell journeys are in the middle of those journeys.

But we then recall Danté's stirring words in the first lines:

"Nel mezzo del cammin di nostra vita/
mi ritrovai per una selva oscura."
"Midway in the journey of our life/
I found myself in a dark wood."
      (Danté, 1970, I, 1–2; Virgil, 2021)

Danté tells us that his midway in the journey that is his life: we have found him fallen into darkness. He readies us for another, a different journey, in fact, a detour. And we recall that the poet Danté was exiled from Florence alleg-edly for corruption, to be executed if he returned.

The traveler, *Danté*, tells us "I was so *full of sleep* at the moment I left the true way" (Au. Italics) (Danté, 1970, I, 11–12; Virgil, 2021). We prepare to hear a journey taken in sleep: a dream/nightmare.

But what journey? He first tries to ascend directly to Paradise. Yet on each of three trials to ascend he is blocked by the leopard (fraud and malice), a lion (violence and bestiality) "raging with hunger," a she-wolf (incontinence) "laden with ever craving and had already caused many to live in sorrow." Being blocked by these three beasts, Danté is accusing himself of bearing, being laden with these sins (*Jeremiah* 5:6). Burdened with these sins, the woe-ful wanderer cannot ascend the hill to heaven.

He laments, "I lost hope of the height."

And then, driven, falling back into his depths, "where the sun is silent," he first hears a voice that is "faint through long silence" then sees its being: Virgil, Danté's poet ideal. Virgil, as if to remind him, identifies himself, "I sang of that just son of Anchises who came from Troy after proud Ilium was burned" (Danté, 1970, I 74–5). Why the long silence, we might wonder? Because few have called upon this guide over the millennia.

The Poet asks the fallen poet, "Why do you not climb the delectable moun-tain . . . of every happiness?"

Danté begins, "You are my master and my author." Then plaintively, "That beast has turned me back, Help me against her." Danté weeps.

Virgil alludes to the start of the journey, go "another way." Then,

Follow me and I will be your guide . . . through an eternal place, where you shall hear despairing shrieks and see the ancient tormented spirits who all bewail the second death . . . if you would then ascend, there shall be a soul worthier than I to guide you.

      (Danté, 1970, I, 112–5)

Listen more to the beginning of this journey.

At first, Danté says he's prepared to follow, and then demurs that he is not Aeneas or Paul, "so I hung back and balked on that dim coast/til thinking had worn out my enterprise" (Danté, 1970, II, 40–41). Danté's thinking had become obsessional so that it interfered with his forward movement.

Virgil crisply responds, "If I have well understood what you say . . . your spirit is beset by cowardice, which often encumbers a man, turning him from the honorable endeavor" (Danté, 1970, II: 45–48). He continues that many men "turn on their course and resolution by imagined perils, as his own shadow turns the frightened horse." The horse *does* see something, but it is a shadow created by himself that frightens him. Virgil knows that this is not a safe journey, but he dissects the fantasy of fear from its reality.

This is a gracious interpretation. First Virgil offers an "out" to Danté: "if I have well understood what you say." Then, the Poet says that this is a common human weakness as one begins an honorable endeavor.

To entice Danté, Virgil reveals who initiated his visit to Danté. The beloved, the deceased Beatrice called to him from Paradise to aid Danté. This woman moves the man.

Why do you lag? Why/
this heart sick hesitation and pale fright/
When three such blessed ladies[12] led from Heaven/
in their concern for you and my own pledge/
of the great good that awaits you has been given?
(Danté, 1970, II 119–23)

Danté's response?

my wilted spirits rose again . . . words have
moved my heart to its first purpose.
My guide my Lord! My master! No lead on:
one will shall serve the two of us in this.
(op cit. II, 127–35)

Virgil does not push or press Danté. He turns, pauses, and waits to continue when Danté is ready to follow. Virgil differs from Aeneas's "guides," whether it is Apollo or shrieking Sibyl.

"Lasciate ogni speranza, voi ch'entrate" (III, 9)
"Abandon all hope, you who enter." (III 8–9)
(Words inscribed over Hell's portal)

What a welcome. It's not screeching Sibyl and the mouths of a thousand caves. It is not the paradoxical words etched above the Oracle of Delphi's cave: "Know thyself." If one knows oneself, one is in less need of an oracle. Instead, we enter beneath an arch of despair: like Auschwitz's "*Arbeit Macht*

Frei" (Work makes (one) free), it is a dark inversion. At the start of Danté's journey, he's told to abandon hope. But, hope, one would think is necessary for an arduous experience such as he feared . . . and would become.

When frightened Danté asks, "What is the meaning of this harsh inscription?"

Virgil clarifies:

> as initiate to novice:
> Here you must put by division of spirit
> and gather our soul against all cowardice.
> This is the place I told you to expect.
> Here you shall pass among the foreign people,
> Souls who have lost the good of intellect.
>
> (III 13–18)

> But Virgil sees that words are not enough, offering his hand "and with a gentle and encouraging smile/he led me through the gate of mystery" (III20–1).

Danté anatomizes Hell and elaborates on Virgil's briefer version where innocent babies are at the periphery, then suicides, and then more felonious characters as one gets deeper. Danté is like the dissected *anatomy* of Hellishness: ten circles, each fiercer, more terrifying than the previous, with a hierarchy of earthly evil. We also learn about the author's, Danté's, value system. And Danté gives payback to some of his unsavory contemporaries and writes their epitaphs. We call this *Schadenfreude*.

Let's do a brief overflight before we microscopically look at a few moments of Danté's terrifying study and the role of his beloved guide.

1. Limbo, for unbaptized or virtuous pagans who did not sin, but did not know Christ: here Danté meets the ancient poets and philosophers— Homer, Horace, Ovid, Lucan, Julius Caesar, Saladin, and Socrates.
2. Lust: Paolo and Francesca who on earth broke adulterous barriers, now hover near each other eternally, never consummating.
3. Gluttony: Ciacco, a contemporary of Danté.
4. Greed: here are two groups—hoarders and lavish spenders. For eternity, they push weights against each other. Many clergymen clustered here.
5. Wrath: two groups crowd the River Styx. On its surface the wrathful battle each other; beneath, the slothful gurgle. A former political enemy, Filippo Argenti is punished here.
6. Heresy: those who countered the Church teachings. Here is one of the more terrifying and poignant encounters. Entombed in eternal flames, Farinata and Cavalcante sit up abruptly, recognizing Danté's Tuscan accent. Danté hesitates, and then engages. In the end, the father only wants to know if his son still lives.

7. Violence: here Danté crosses three rings:

   A. Outer ring of violence *against neighbors* who are submerged in a river of blood;
   B. Middle ring of violence *against oneself* (recall Virgil's place for these): they are transformed into gnarled trees and bushes, consumed by harpies (perhaps a model for Ovid's *Metamorphosis*);
   C. Inner ring of *violence against god, art, and nature:* here are blasphemers, sodomites, and users in a desert of burning sand and fiery rain. Intriguingly, Danté discovers his former mentor, Brunetto Latini.

8. Fraud: divided into ten ditches (*bogias*) each for different frauds: seducers, flatterers, diviners, hypocrites, thieves, and others. Perhaps to our surprise, Jason appears (Surprised? Ah, but he did abandon his wife Medea.); Ulysses appears (Yes, the fine *polytropos*, "many turning" man, deceiver.) and of course, popes and politics.

9. Treachery: frozen in different layers of a lake of their own tears, the worst are frozen up to their eyes. Listen to the excruciating detail:
   "faces upturned. The very weeping there prevents their weeping and the grief . . . turns inward to increase the agony, for the first tear form a knot and, like a crystal visor, fill all the cup beneath the eyebrow" (XXXIII, 93 ff).

10. Severe treachery: the three selected are Judas, Brutus, and Cassius (Paired Betrayers of Caesar) in the maw of Lucifer's crunching jaws.

And to escape Hell, Danté clasps onto panting Virgil's neck, as he climbs down Lucifer's "shaggy flanks . . . matted hair, and the frozen crusts, . . . where the thigh turns just at the thick of the haunch . . . so that I thought I was returning to Hell again" (XXXIV 72–81). "Panting Virgil," yes, even the great Virgil must exert himself to protect his charge. But they reach intermediate Purgatory. This is no exit such as Virgil's elegant (if false) Dream Gate of ivory.

Danté offers an obvious reason for selecting Virgil as his guide: Virgil is his master Poet, albeit in Latin. While Danté the poet wrote in Latin for his earlier work, for this masterpiece, when he is exiled from Florence and threatened with execution should he return, Danté turned to his mother tongue, Italian. And he writes in terza rhyme, the everyday patois of Italian.

But a second reason for selecting Virgil emerges as we read. Virgil knows the territory of Hell; he's been on this journey before, with Aeneas. He is an experienced guide to the dangers that lie ahead. And he has said (via Juno):

Flectere si nuques superos, Acheronta movebo
If I cannot move the higher powers, I will move the infernal regions.
                    (Aeneid, VII, 312 and Freud, 1900 inscription).

Danté will move us further; after moving the infernal regions, he will take us to the higher powers, step by excruciating step.

Let us take a few scenes from *The Inferno* to learn from Danté what he is gathering and from whom he learns on this perilous, terrifying voyage.

Hesitations

The Odyssey is replete with weepings including Odysseus' and Telemachus bawling on each other's shoulders until Apollo almost pries them apart with a demand for battle and blood. Aeneas also has his weepings, such as his display to Dido, his father's tears upon seeing his son alive, and Aeneas' response, "his face streaming tears." In contrast, *The Inferno* is replete with faintings, and Danté's *and* Virgil's pallor. This humanizes both Danté and Virgil. Overall, we see that the poet Danté presents Virgil to us as a transformed, more humanistic, and humane ghost/man/poet compared to the Virgil who wrote of "Arms and the man I sing. *Armo Virunque cano*" (I, 1).

Fainting, paling, and hesitations are markers along this journey. We can study Danté's hesitations to learn why he stops, and pauses, what he fears, and possibly what we learn about him and his guide at each moment of reluctance.

Danté's first hesitation we've mentioned earlier: when he first hears Virgil's indistinct voice, he fears it is a shadow coming to torment him further. Then Danté reveals something of himself when he says, "You are my true master," his ideal.

Virgil takes this opportunity to foretell Danté's journey:

> for your own good, I think it well you follow me and I will be your guide. And lead you forth through an eternal place. There you shall see the ancient spirits tried in endless pains and hear their lamentation as each bemoans the second death of souls. Next you shall see upon a burning mountain, souls in fire and yet content in fire knowing that . . . they yet will mount into the blessed choir. To which, if is stair you wish to climb a worthier spirit shall be sent to guide you. With her shall I leave you for the King of Time.
>
> (I, 105–17)

Hell, Purgatory, Heaven in a sweeping breath.

Danté's second hesitation, mentioned earlier, is when he demurs that he is not Paul or Aeneas, how dare he proceed on this path? Virgil's response: he tells Danté implicitly that he does not need to be in league with Saints or Heroes to engage in this (dream) journey. Anyone can undertake this voyage provided he faces his normal cowardice. And Eros (Beatrice) will move Danté to overcome his hesitation. The historical driving force for a man's life journey was Fate (Heraclitus, Homer), which was replaced by the search for Truth (Plato, Gorgias). Then Aristotle offers Tragedy as a vicarious driving force to purify the soul. Virgil is the first major poet of sentimental love, emphasizing the unity of character and fate. Danté saw "love as a mediator of divine wisdom" that could confer faith, knowledge, and renewal (Auerbach, 1954, 27). "Renewal" is another way we can think of all the voyages above—Odysseus, Aeneas, and Danté—for they all emerge from Hell almost reincarnated, renewed, at least in the soul, if not literally in flesh.

Danté's third hesitation is at Hell's gate. But, unlike Aeneas, it is not some screeching banshee Sibyl and the mouths of 1,000 caves that howl at him. It is the quiet inscription to abandon all hope. Virgil offers a lesson here: Danté must "put aside division of spirit/gather your soul against all cowardice." This journey, we will learn, is about unifying Danté's inner self, in order to overcome cowardice within; in order to better his life, to reach Paradise. And Virgil offers more than his words and he extends his hand "with a gentle and encouraging smile" (III, 20–1).

The fourth and fifth hesitations are at and in Charon's boat to cross the River Styx. First, it is an external power that pauses Danté's journey: Charon won't take a living soul across, citing the violence done by Hercules (beheading Cerebrus) and others. Virgil steps in, waves off his objection, and reassures Charon that Danté will not harm, only observe. Then, in the laden boat, Danté, upon hearing the cries of pain of those on the other shore—infants ripped by death from the breast, innocents—faints. We learn something of Danté and his sensibilities. And that he may have to develop more inner strength to observe the severe punishments meted out to others in hell, even if deserved punishments. Pity (a characteristic of Aeneas, *pietas*) must be complemented by understanding. *Tout comprendre, c'est tout pardonner; All that is understood, is pardoned.*[13]

In Limbo, Danté is among the five great poets. What is this? What "gives" here? Why relegate the great (pre-Christian) poets to Hell at all? We can but speculate. The poets represent the purity of reason. But as we progress, we learn with Danté that *Reason must be fused, or infused with Eros*, passion, to bring us higher in life. The myth of Psyche and Eros embodies this ideal union.

Sixth hesitation: gazing down into the abyss of Hell. Here, Virgil pales:

Death-pale, the poet spoke: "Now let us go into the blind world . . . I will lead you and you and shall follow."

Danté, alarmed at Virgil's pallor, responds:

How can I go this way when you who are my strength, in doubt turn pale with terror?

The pain of these below . . . drowns the color from my face for *pity* and leaves this pallor you *mistake* for fear . . . Now let us go, for a long road awaits us.

(Danté IV, 19–22; My emphasis)

Here, Virgil clarifies: Danté correctly *sees* Virgil's pallor but *misinterprets* its internal meaning.

At the seventh moment for pause, Minos orders Danté back. They are about to enter the circle of those who betrayed reason by their appetites (impulses), particularly sexual incontinence.[14] Virgil intercedes: "This is not your concern, it is his fate to enter every door" (V, 20–2). Virgil tells us and Danté: first that it is Danté's concern that will drive us forward; and second that Danté is fated to enter every door of Hell. This contrasts, as you recall, with Aeneas who upon asking about the screams emerging from Tartarus is told that he cannot enter there, but Sibyl will inform him of those torments. Not here; here Danté will enter every door and draw his own conclusions.

The eighth hesitation is marked by a shift between Virgil and Danté. In general, Virgil as a guide will point to things for Danté to see but permits Danté to draw conclusions from the scene. That is, first the sensual (sight) is used by the mind to create new knowledge. Second, Virgil is pressing Danté now, not only to draw conclusions but also to "see" what he believes he is not prepared to see. Perceiving the adulterous Francesca and Paolo, Danté feels he can't look at them. Virgil suggests calling to them. When he does call on the lovers, sees them, and then listens to their story, Danté swoons. But he recovers, now on his own to enter the circle of gluttony, guarded by three-headed Cerberus, ever-famished to consume whatever wants to pass. Filling his mouth with filth, Virgil wordlessly passes on. Danté shows concern about the future of these gluttons. Virgil offers some tempered hope:

As for these souls, though they can never soar,/
To true perfection, still in the new time/
They will be nearer it than they were before.
(Danté, VI, 106–8)

Even in the depths of hell, as long as one's sins are not to the depths below the treachery of Judas, for instance, there is hope . . . with time.

Within the first few circles, with the first eight hesitations, we have passed desire, fear, and hopelessness, counterbalanced by some hope and more significantly for Danté, some insights into the human soul, particularly his.

There's more, far more to this Hellish journey with associated enlightenment for Danté. But we have covered the fundamentals of Virgil as a guide, a far more humane and instructive guide than Aeneas had, certainly than Odysseus. And we hear how Danté has humanized his dear master poet. We hear Danté's insights and how he achieves them with Virgil's support and encouragement. *Virgil believes in Danté more than the poet believes in himself.* And we see the resonating interaction between Danté and Virgil. Let us turn to comparing the hellish voyages of these three—the heroes, Odysseus, and Aeneas, and the downcast poet who becomes heroic in the course of his Infernal voyage.

Denouement

Saul Bellow said that any good author takes up the challenges of previous great author and tries to address them (Personal Communication, 1972). So too with Aeneas and later Danté: they build upon Homer and later, Danté upon Virgil. Millennia may separate them, but it is if they are in dialogue or at least responds to each other, as if they were colleagues, contemporaries, and fellow laborers in wordsmithing.

What Are the Basic Similarities?

All three recognize that somewhere in the midst of a life's journey, one must descend to an underworld in order to travel not only further but to one's home. All three benefit from learning from those who dwell in the Underworld. For Odysseus, it is primarily the gender-shifted Tiresias, although we will be moved by his encounter with Odysseus' mother (what he learns of his home's status), and from his brief tete-a-tete with Achilles. Odysseus lauds the heroism-unto-death of Achilles; Achilles would prefer to be a living servant to being a dead king of the dead (Freud, 1925, 294). This poignant remark stands out in bold after the slashing, stabbing, warring *Iliad*, and the *Odyssey's* ending of mayhem; Achilles' moving comment returns us to the beginning of Odysseus' life journey, a journey that he was so reluctant to embark upon that he feigned madness for a month before Agamemnon caught him in the act and prevailed upon Odysseus to start this two decade's long voyage.

Recall that Tiresias, that blind seer who will offer prophetic wisdom. Recall his tragic life trajectory. Seeing two snakes copulating, he is punished by being transformed from a man to a woman. Later, seeing two other snakes copulating, he is transformed back into a man. But his tragedy is compounded by Jove and Juno's fractious disagreement. They can't agree whether man or woman has more pleasure in sex: Jove, that serial adulterer, insists it is women; Juno, men. They agree to consult Tiresias as he has experienced both sides of sexual life. He says that definitely women enjoy sex more. In payment for his honesty, furious Juno blinds him.[15] Unable to reverse his wife's curse, Jove grants Tiresias the ability to "see" the future. This multiply-cursed man, now a ghost, will grant Odysseus his vision of the future.

We've already noted that Odysseus is educated by Circé, his second seductress, who sends him to the Underworld: "There is another journey which you have got to take before you can sail homewards . . . to the house of Hades of dread Proserpine."[16] She puts aft winds into his sails to navigate his trip. Odysseus needs Circé's help and guidance: his navigation to her is fraught and roundabout. Landing on Aeolus, the King of Winds entertained him for a month in exchange for Odysseus' rhetorical account of the Trojan War. Then, Aeolus "flayed me a prime ox-hide to hold the ways the roaring winds, which he shut up in the hide as in a sack" (Homer, X, 1). For nine days and nights, they sailed well until, as Odysseus nodded off at the tiller, his men became suspicious that this sack contained riches that he would not share with them. Undoing the sack, releasing the contending winds, undoes their journey. Fierce winds bore them back to Aeolus, who reacts with astonishment, then fear and anger: "Vilest of mankind, get you gone at once . . . him whom heaven hates . . . abhorred of heaven" (Homer, X, 200).

At their next landing, the giant Laestrygonians "speared them (his men) like fishes and took them home to eat them." Only then could they land at Circé's enchanted island. All these surrealistic experiences could have been nightmarishly dreamt.

Even so, Odysseus' Hell entrance is relatively simple: two trenches a cubit each crosswise, then filled with honey and milk, then wine, then water, and then sprinkled with white barley meal. After Odysseus' fervent prayers, he sacrifices two sheep, running their blood into the trenches; blood opens the throats of Tiresias and other ghosts.

And prophesize Tiresias does: a long, tumultuous return home, his ship, and all his men destroyed; kill all the suitors; carry an oar to "a country where the people have never heard of the sea and do not even mix salt with their food . . . nothing about ships and oars that are as the wings of a ship" (Homer, XI, 236). And for Odysseus? "Death shall come to you from the sea and your life shall ebb away very gently when you are full of years and peace find and your people shall bless you" (Homer, XI, 238).

The last phrase is the closest we come to the future generations.

Virgil carries us much further into the prophesied future, as spoken by Father Anchises. He gives more weight to Aeneas's labored return to a new shore, a new home. And his father articulates both Aeneas's and heirs' roles: the art of rule.

Of Danté, we have more hope than prophesy. While he too realizes that he must endure an underworld journey, we perceive differences. Danté is not hero, no Odysseus, no Aeneas. He is but a poet, perhaps even a minor poet who has been writing in rarified Latin. Yes, this poet is exiled from his home and we suspect yearns to return. But his voyage is to an ultimate home: the arms of his Beatrice and hence, the entrance to Paradise. His first task for the poet Danté is to adopt his mother tongue, Italian, even before the character Danté embarks on his journey.

Let us expand on the differences among these three Underworld wanderers or voyagers not only to differentiate them but also to apply them to psychoanalytic work, and more importantly, to our work with the aftermath of the Hell of October 7.

We see significant differences comparing the fourteenth-century CE Danté to the circa 30 CE Virgil to the circa 700 BCE Odyssey. Odysseus, as we've seen yearns to return to his old home, although his gods and war delay him by two decades. As do Calypso and Circé. Borges argues that Odysseus as a "true" Greek hero is unchanged from the beginning to the end: he is *poly-tropos*, many-formed, devious, clever, and wiley from his "horse" days to his disguised suitor-slaying day. By this, Borges means unchanged in character. Mendelsohn (Personal Communication, 2023) suggests that we might see different aspects of Odysseus upon returning home, at least the contemporary reader may: does he interact differently with Penelope? Was Penelope "on" to his disguised true self as Odysseus? We can debate this; however, we do not suggest that there is character change, perhaps some transformation revealing a different conformation as the shoulder-weeping father or softened husband. But in the end, it is the wiley, ruthless Odysseus who reclaims his turf and wife by slaughtering 108 suitors and hanging their maidservants, even as he was prepared to throttle his old nursemaid as she was washing his feet should she say his name. We recall the touching scene as his son finally recognizes him, but this may have been no different than the Odysseus refusing to go to battle for another's purloined wife, Helena, when he had a newborn son and wife.

We can read the Odysseus voyage through hell and return to his old home as an example of how some patients turn to psychoanalysis. They hope to return to a time, a place before their years of vicissitudes, a form of regression to (at least imagined) equilibrium. They ascribe responsibility for their vicissitudes to external powers—gods or people (like Odysseus' men, who all *had* to die for their transgressions and jeopardize his voyage). They do not see their contributions to their miseries, even at the end of their voyage. Their journey through the dream underworld reveals no significant insights but strengthens the yearning to go back to the ("unchanged") home they left. We, observers from the outside, may see that after years of absence, the home is different—the Telemachus son is grown, albeit a bit unmoored, seeking his father; the Penelope is still yearning for her husband, although she shows her mettle by deceiving the suitors with her weaving/unweaving; and the father is worn down, bereft, sleeping outside in his vineyard. We see the changes; Odysseus is inured to many of these.

Aeneas offers a different underworld voyage that can apply to others who come for and are guided through treatment. He knows that his homeland is destroyed. He bears his past (his father) on his shoulders, his future by the hand (his son), and loses his wife (to death). He remains accompanied by his cohort of men, not "losing" them as did Odysseus. He has different peer relatedness. He knows that he must find a new home but not how to navigate there, for he doesn't know where *there* is. His father prophesies that Aeneas will know his new homeland by watching his famished son eat his "plate." In his Underworld voyage, his "guide" presents as a maddened, shrieking, threatening, bucking Sibyl who won't let him enter, until Aeneas softens her first with emollient words, then, with a gift, a Golden Bough and offers for sacrifices in the future. Yes, the fee helps lubricate the analysis. Winnicott (1974) might have seen this as a form of "hate" in the countertransference. Sibyl advises him along the way but warns him that the most hellish areas (we might say, of inner life), the Tartarus of torture, he cannot enter, although she will describe it to him. We will contrast this with Virgil's reprimand of Minos, who wants to bar Danté's way. Aeneas protects his men, as they accompany and aid him. But even as he arrives and finds new love (beyond his fantasied Dido who loves him more than he her), he awakens to find he must battle for his new wife and his new home. He is now psychologically armed for battle; from his father he learns the far future, his heirs, and the reasons for his struggle now and in the future. These patients feel compelled—by trauma such as the fall of Troy, or by close others (Dido) who press them to seek cures.

Danté, those five letters that make other writers tremble. As mentioned, Auerbach considered Danté the greatest of all writers. We need not debate that here; let us simply accept that he was a great writer. But also, Danté, as Bellow stated, built upon the success of his predecessors, particularly Homer and Virgil, in accounts of Hell at least.

Danté, unlike Odysseus and Aeneas, sees himself as having lived up to his mid-life, not as fully as he should have. He is in a dark wood mostly of his own making. Of course, like many in mid-life crises, he tries to ascend directly to Paradise. But he is impeded: in the poem it is the lion, the she-wolf, the leopard. But we know from Danté's era that these represented *inner* human weakness—ravenous hunger, envy, and pride. And Danté does not state that these are external gods, as do the Greeks, as does Sibyl, who plague him; we understand that these are very human, inner weaknesses, that he must overcome. Somehow. But not alone. Danté, like those few mentioned in the Aeneid in the Sibyl's commentary, has that fiery inner desperate need to seek repair of his self. When Danté finds a guide (chooses, accepts), it is his ego ideal, the long-dead, too long-silent Virgil. And Virgil reveals that there is another "way" to get to Paradise; one that is treacherous, fearsome. And Virgil offers to accompany him. Virgil's relationship with Danté is a model for psychoanalysis; he takes him by layers of increasing depth, primitivity, and danger. He points out things to observe and waits to see if Danté is prepared to observe. He allows Danté to draw his own conclusions. And the poet Danté builds a hierarchy of evil, of human weaknesses: the adulterous Francesca and Paolo are closer to the innocent babes who died without baptism, are closer to the admired poets who lived before Christ, and are far removed from gluttonous popes and bishops and certainly ten circles distant from the trio of treachery—Judas, Brutus, and Cassius. Early on, Virgil offers another reason for Danté to move through Hell; he is sent by the trio of Beatrice, Lucy, and Rachel to bring Danté to Heaven. What waits for him after this arduous journey is the truest love. It is not only a new "home" but the home in the arms of his beloved.

Danté also goes into great detail beyond the visuals of Odysseus' Hell and certainly Aeneas. Recall that when Aenius hears the greatest of torments, the Sybil will not take him there to *see* their suffering; she will only tell him of this. But Danté sees all the suffering in *The Inferno*—burning Ferrananté or Cavalcanté bolt upright from his tomb; Ugolino gnawing at Bishop Rugierro's skull for eternity, or the three greatest of traitors—Brutus and Cassius gripped by their feet and Judas, head in Satan's jaws—being eternally whipped and ripped apart in Satan's teeth. What is "seen" cannot be unseen. And we only hear or read Danté's word-painting of these sufferings; still we cannot "unsee" them. Danté set the standards for Western (Christian) Hell, including the visualized eternal torments of the body. In our final account of Hell, October 7th, 2023 Israel, we will learn how what is seen cannot be unseen. But let us finish our tours of antique Hells with some thoughts about psychoanalysis, one method to climb out of personal Hells, a guide aiding our ascent.

Bettelheim (Person Communication, 1968) taught that there are three resonating stages of psychoanalysis:

1. "Look at what bad things were done to me" (by my mother/father/sister/brother/others).
2. "*That* is why I suffer today."
3. "But why do you continue to suffer when you no longer live with my mother/father/sister/brother/others?" The Analyst might ask.

Many analysands get stuck resonating between stages one and two. It is the analyst's task to help them examine stage three, and their contribution to maintaining their inner misery. Danté comes closest to achieving the third phase of self-analysis.

These three underworld journeys describe not only the underworld of our oneiric sleep lives, and our dreams but also different pathways to enter treatment and different "homes" to find solace. For those survivors of October 7, we understand the resonating between "Look what was done to me and those whom I love." And "This is why I suffer." How do we help them achieve the third level of living: "Why do you perpetuate your suffering today? How do we help you emerge from that true Hell? What is the future life to build?"

Now we turn to October 7th, the undreamed nightmare of a people, an earthquake with ongoing after tremors.

Notes

1 Such as when wily Helena tries to lure the soldiers out of the Trojan horse by imitating each soldier's wife's voice.
2 In *Odysseus in Vietnam*, Jonathan Shay, moving and persuasively argues that the US soldiers in Vietnam experienced much of what Homer describes of the Greeks and Trojans. He writes an equally persuasive case of US soldiers returning to America in his *Ulysses in America*.
3 Generous but gracious treatment of the guest.
4 Daniel Mendelsohn offered this insight into gorging, satiation, restraint, and murder (Personal Communication, 2023).
5 In the later Ovid *Metamorphosis* (2004), sexual transgressions result in inanimate or beastly unhuman body transformations.
6 We recall that Freud also initiate this dream studies after his father's death.
7 We will note that Freud too entered *his* Irma dream world via *her* nasal cavities ("die Nasenhøle"). We can speculate on the connection to entering a woman's other "hole."
8 We hear an echo of Oedipus.
9 Pheobus, "bright one," is an epithet of Apollo, generally when he is identified with the sun. Of course, the Virgil poet would find a place among the Elysian Fields for poets.
10 In that famous scene, the father, Anchises, is connected to Aeneas' son who eats his plate: Aeneas is the pivot between the past prophesy and the present realization.
11 Whether the home he returns to is precisely the home to this past is a more complex issue for another time. Borges (2002) claims that Odysseus returns unchanged from the beginning of the epic, and by this, he means his character is unchanged. But there are hints that other aspects of his inner life may have transformed.

12 Beatrice, Lucy, and Rachel.
13 We are translating *pardonner* as pardoned, rather than "forgiven." Some sins cannot be forgiven, as we will see in Danté's progress, or as we know from horrid, bestial acts such as the October 7 Hamas infant/child/civilian murders, mutilations, and celebration of horrors. A Hamas terrorist GoPro's himself cutting a fetus out of a living woman's belly, and then kills them both; there is no punishment in Hell severe enough for eternity for such a beast.
14 We note here that this post-Christ poem replays the pre-Christ Ovid's and Virgil's punishments for sexual "incontinence" or transgressions.
15 No good deed goes unpunished, these gods might insist.
16 The women of *The Odyssey* send men on treacherous, long-duration journey from Helena to Circé to Athena (trying to bring Odysseus home), to the ever-faithful Penelope, whose magnetic attraction pulls Odysseus homeward. This is a subject for another time.

References

Auerbach, E. 1954. *Mimesis: The Representation of Reality in Western Literature.* Princeton University Press.
Borges, J. 2002. *Ficciones*. Penguin.
Danté. 1970. *The Inferno,* Tr. Ciardi, 1–2. Rutgers University Press.
Freud, S. 1900. *The Interpretation of Dreams*. epigraph. Hogarth Press.
Freud, S. 1925. *Inhibitions, Symproms and Anxiety*. Hogarth Press.
Homer. 1990. *Odyssey,* Tr. R. Fagles. Penguin.
Ovid, Metamorphosis. 2004. Tr. David Raeburn. Penguin.
Virgil, Aeneid. 2021. Tr. Shadi Barsch. Random House.
Winnicott, D. W. 1974. *The Maturational Processes and The Facilitating Environment*. IUP.

2 Hell on Earth

What's Seen Cannot Be Unseen

What you will read below challenges us. Can we accept the former slave, later philosopher, Terence's declaration, *"Homo sum, humani nihil a me alienum puto."* "Human am I, (hence) nothing human is alien to me." Millennia later, Primo Levy said of his Auschwitz sojourn (with dismay?) "If this is a man." "Se questo è un uomo."[1] Listen.

A humanoid—human in appearance, satanic within—fucks a woman from behind. Whenever she screams, he stabs her with a knife in her back, into her lungs, collapsing them. Another humanoid lops off this woman's breast and tosses it about until he discards it. In the end, a humanoid shoots her in the head.

One humanoid holds a mother from behind and grabs her hair to force her to watch. Another humanoid throws her living baby into an oven to be burnt to death.

One humanoid duct-tapes a pregnant woman's mouth, stifling her screams. Another humanoid holds her from behind. Humanoid Satan cuts out her living fetus. Then both mother and baby are shot in the head.

Many Satans—yes Satans revealed, as their actions destroy humanoid appearances—fuck-rape a woman . . . no several women. They keep fuck-raping one until her pelvis is shattered and she dies from exsanguination. Or they shoot her to death when done with her. One Satan fucks and then shoots her in the head before he calmly zips his prick cover.

Satans tie a father and child back-to-back with wire and then shoot the pair to death.

Satans grab people, sling them over a motorcycle or throw them into a truck and take them to Hell, Satan's home, the Hell that these beast-Satans have just created on Earth. Wherever the Satans' hooves trod, Hell follows; nothing lives after they pass.

A Satan drives nails into a woman's vagina. Satans shoot men in the genitals, in the face, and women in their breasts. Sex organs seem a preoccupation for these Satans, something to be attacked and destroyed. In Ovid, many metamorphoses—transformations from humans to objects—are experienced *after* a sexual transgression. Here, Hell on Earth, Satans transform humans into death, the ultimate degradation, the end of vitality, the end of any hope.

DOI: 10.4324/9781003618690-3

Heads are lopped off; not with a quick machete, but arduously sawed away with a knife, or hacked with a gardening spade. Limbs are amputated and discarded roadside. Into a bomb shelter filled with children, Satans toss grenades.

All this was meticulously filmed with GoPros by the Satanic beasts to document their achievements, to show the world what they can do. One Satan in the guise of a human kills a person, and then uses the human's phone to call his mother and father and brag that he's killed ten Jews with his bare hands—he shows his bloody hands to prove this. His parents praise him. We can hear the audio of the call, his excitement, and their pride. Another Satan phones his buddy to brag that he's brought home a living "whore," a Jewess, and a "noble steed." We guess he'll "ride" her. He perhaps is alluding to Mohammed's kidnapping of teenage Jewess, Tzofiya bat Huyyay ("re-christened" as Safiyya bint Huyayy) in 628 after Mohammed slaughtered her family in the Battle of Khaybar. Wikipedia politely says she was "widowed" without stating that she was "widowed" by the Moslem marauders. Muhammed ordered Tzofiya's Jewish husband tortured with hot steel burning chest until near death and then beheaded. Tzofiya became Muhammed's fourth "wife." She is "worshipped" in Islam. Mohammed died four years later.

Ecclesiastes begins, *"Eyn Chadash tachat ha' shemesh,"* "Nothing new under the sun," especially for Moslem marauders.

At least Danté portrayed the Satanic tortures in diabolical forms: Satan himself has three heads; others have forked tongues or tails; another has six limbs, two of the middle ones transforming into a penis. Hieronymous Bosch two centuries later portrayed visual devils, with appurtenances of forked tails and tongues and hooves. But the October 7th Satans look have the appearance of being human or at least humanoid. Their actions and their glee in their murderous, torturing mayhem reveal their inner evil. Even the Nazis did not enact some of these monstrous torments (although some of their minions—Czech or Ukrainian adjuncts—tried hard to outdo the SS).

I live in earthquake country, California, a few miles from the San Andreas fault. We learn that after an earthquake, prepare for aftershocks.

Aftershocks?

As I talk with my colleague, Professor Gal Meiri by WhatsApp, I hear the bombings of Beersheva, where he lives. A playground is hit. And also the bombings in Gaza. During our talk, one of his two sons calls to tell him that he is serving in the West Bank but has noticed that he may be called up to Gaza. Gal asks me, "When one son was in Gaza and the other sent to the north against Hezbollah, how am I to serve as a psychiatrist, as a physician, when I am worried about my sons?"

A student talks with me by Facetime from the cafeteria of his university in Herziliya. A student, yes. Also, he has finished seven years in Shayetet (Navy Seals) as have his three brothers. Finished until October 7, he then restarted. He is asking me to plan a program to transition warriors into students—how to diminish the hypervigilance, the loss of concentration, and the "scanning" of second-floor University windows for snipers. Then we are interrupted, he must get to the shelter as Hezbollah is bombing his town. A few minutes later, he returns (I am relieved), picking up where we left off. Yes, how to transition from soldier to student, but while in the midst of war.

Shocks and aftershocks? Dr. Sapir is a psychiatric resident who was on duty at Soroka Hospital in Beersheva on October 7. That morning at 8:00 a.m. still at the Hospital, she can't reach her husband and two sons in their Kibbutz Erez, a border community, which she later learned was under attack. She texts her fellow residents to get someone to cover her shift at Soroka so she can drive to Erez to find her family. (It is still 8:00 a.m. on October 7, before the government announces the attacks on the border communities.) A Bedouin resident texts that he lives closest and will cover.

At Soroka Hospital, the helipad, once a site for excitement, now is used almost daily for critically wounded soldiers from Gaza. Where once faculty gathered at the windows to watch incoming helicopters, now they have reactions of fear, apprehension, and dread at the sound of the choppers.

At Beit Tzipporah, the after-school program for Ethiopian children funded by Elie Wiesel and named after his sister murdered in Auschwitz, when the *azakah*, the red alert alarm for incoming missiles screams, the children begin to cry. Why? They do not fear for themselves. Rather they fear for their father, or uncle, or brother serving in Gaza. The principal asks for help. Can we help the children?

My colleague Haim Belmaker, a renowned neuropsychiatrist, and I are talking on WhatsApp. How can we plan a return visit for me to continue consulting in Israel? I mention I want to come for a longer time but with my four children and wife. Haim, a father of five, a grandfather, cautions that this would not be a good time to bring children who have not become accustomed to air raids screams, bombs falling about them. Not a good time (for my children). I internally resist this. *Kol Yisrael Averim Zeh Be-Zeh*.

I am reminded of my friend Shlomi Ravid of Glil Yam Kibbutz in the center of Herzilyah. During the second Intifada, American parents would call asking if it were safe for their teen children to visit. Shlomi would think to himself (but not say to them) not safe, not safe for my children either. When Shlomi's seven-year-old son, knowing that his father was a tank commander would climb the tank monument saying he too wanted to be a tank soldier, Shlomi and his wife prayed that he never would have to serve. A prayer denied by the enduring enemies of the Jews.

These are aftershocks. How do we "treat" the responses to October 7, when the evocations of war continue? This is not new territory for soldiers. Grinker, Zahava Solomon, and others have paved the way. But what about children? We will discover new approaches here.

"From Hell to Eternity" was my initial provocative title for this book; it challenges us to critical thinking. For, how can there be an eternity of future: the sun will flame out, like every other star; or the earth will flameout by the hand of man and unless Elon Musk can establish mankind on Mars beforehand, humankind—god's best and worst creation—will be gone? If ever there needed to be proof of a Death Instinct, a Death Drive, *ecce homo*, "Here's the man"!

But there is another "eternity" I suggest. An "eternity" that my children grasp. It is a dangling bright future before them; the past—their predecessor—is a prelude to their own lives. My 11-year-old designs ever faster, ever sleeker cars with two friends; my nine-year-old hopes that if he attends Stanford, he'll still be able to play for the Warriors; my seven-year-old looks forward to a more advanced Lego set or a wristwatch with dancing arms, and my two and half year old greets each morning with extended arms seeking an embrace and only then, a bottle of milk. These are their psychological eternities, hopeful expectations that the future will continue like this.

The United States for much of its history has been a land of hope, streets paved with gold . . . until recently. In the past decades, some segments of Americans have focused on and condemned the United States as victimizing, and hence if not evil, at least needs to be more than criticized, even destroyed. Feminists damn the penile-dominated country; some Blacks seek reparations (discounting the tens of thousands of Northern soldiers dead in the battle against slavery; then tens of thousands who marched with MLK); some Islamists shout "Death to America." And as both Hamas and Iran have proclaimed, these words—"Death to America" or "From the River to the Sea"—have consequences, have potential destructive energy behind them. Believe them.

Israel's "eternity" has been on a short leash. "*Hatikvah*," the national anthem means "hope." It sings that Jews have hoped to return for 2,000 years. (Most nations, even religions are not as old as this Jewish hope to return to native land.) And return Jews did. But, since 1948, specific "wars" punctuate Jewish history in Israel—1956, 1967, 1973, Lebanon I and II, the first Gaza war, now October 7 and April 13 (Iran's missile barrage). In fact, Israel has been harassed with attacks, brutal murders of children and others almost continuously from the 1920s. Little eternity here, unless we consider this an eternity of surrounding animosity, an eternal hell created by man.

Moses selected a "prince" from each of the 12 tribes to scout out the Land. They returned hiking the kilometer height of Qadesh Barnea, two bearing grape vines on their shoulders, but ten reporting a hostile populace: a land that eats its inhabitants, Israelites will be like insects before these giants.

Insects and giants could be a footnote. But it deserves more. When Eli Cohen, the Jewish spy in Syria, was about to be hung by the Syrians, his last words were to look out upon the Land of Israel and proclaim "From here you look like giants."

Moses, standing on the precipice of Qadesh Barnea, scanning the desolate shaley scarp at the Egyptian border northward, proclaimed "This a land of milk and honey." When I biked up Qadesh Barea and looked out, I thought, "Quite an imagination this Moses had." For what did this mean—milk and honey—then? For milk, at that time, one didn't have cows in sheds waiting to be milked; one didn't have constructed hives with garbed beekeepers protected from stings. Instead, milk came from the wandering shepherd with his goats and sheep; honey from the predecessors of Pooh Bear, climbing trees to feed from hives. This blessing was mixed.

Moses made a strategic decision; listened to the ten negative princes, cast aside Caleb and Joshua's praises of the land. Elderly Moses chose to guide the Jewish nation on a 40-year trek through the desert; long enough for the enslaved elders to die; and a new, desert-hardened generation to enter the land, a tough country. Even Moses died without entering the land.

Forty years is not an eternity . . . except for the generation that died out, they met their eternity. But the next great exiles of Jews, 2,000 years after the Roman conquest, felt almost eternal. Roman soldiers on horseback complained that Jerusalem was running with so much Jewish blood—to the horses' chests, that they had trouble slogging through the town. Yet Jews kept praying to return.

And return they did, again perhaps hardened by two millennia of exiles, pogroms, intermittently thriving among strangers in strange lands and being murdered, raped, exiled by them.

When 1848 brought great births of nations in Europe, the Jews were left isolated; no home for them . . . there. The Israeli national hymn, "Hatikva," "the hope," looks forward from two millennia of exile. Written by Imber, living in a Polish, then Galician, now Ukrainian town, in 1877, the poem was set to a Romanian folk tune by Shmuel Cohen in 1887 in Petah Tikva, after Imber moved to Israel. Shimon Peres, former President of Israel, remarked that without hope, there would be no Israel. And hope points us to the future, if not eternity, then part-way there, incrementally.

October 7, 2023, then April 13, 2024, changed that. Changed us. Israel is a small gnat for massive Iran and its proxies: a hard (nuclear) smack and Israel is smashed, wiped out. Now the question for Israeli parents is whether there is a future (not an eternity) for their children; can they feel hope for the future?

This chapter follows the first three ancient "heroes": from descent to (internal) enlightenment to ascent of Odysseus, Aeneus, and Danté. How can we ascend from the unspeakable horrors of October 7 and what could have been on April 13? We recall Winnicott's first response to the British government on how to help children. First, DWW the practical pediatrician, said, keep them safe. Then we can take care of the rest. Keep them safe is the military (and perhaps diplomatic) remedy. The rest is for people like us, psychoanalysts, and parents to build.

What have we learned from these three Antique heroes, these predecessors? All descended with some reluctance. Danté portrays this more clearly. He, in misery, in despair, tries to ascend directly to Paradisical Light. He is tossed down by three sins. In Danté, there are three beasts. But also in Danté we hear that they represent internal sins from which he must be cured. This cure occurs via a guided voyage through Hell, a guide who has gone this Hellish route before, who knows both its dangers and its earnings. Danté learns from the sufferings of others; he has more observing Ego available than those who suffer fire or ice.

What can we do with this here?

There are no "sins" that merited the punishment of those tortured and slaughtered on October 7. We can quote Marc Antony's final lines in Shakespeare's *Julius Caesar* "My heart is there, in the coffin with Caesar/and I must pause till it come back to me." Like Antony, we need to feel and recognize that our hearts are buried with the dead of October 7 and the dead soldiers in Gaza. But we must like Antony and recognize that our hearts must come back to us: to choose life.

Israel was made vulnerable by its self-destructive, implacable, animosity that thousands, even tens of thousands of Israelis demonstrated in streets *against other Israelis* for months preceding October 7. This "sin" per Talmud is called *Sinat Chinam*, which I'll discuss further. It translates literally as "free hate," but means the (unfounded) hatred of brother against brother, which the rabbis said "caused" the fall of Jerusalem, the Temple, to the Romans two millennia ago. We even recall that Queen Shlomtzion's two sons were in battle with each other over who would become king, a battle that we can recognize among the contenders for prime minister today. This made (and will make) Israel and Israelis appear weak before its enemies; and led their enemies to believe we could be rent, ripped apart. What to learn?

I write this even as some of the ˆ*verbrendte*, "burning" angry Israeli men and women prior to October 7th, return to the streets with animosity toward fellow Jews.

Another "sin" was that the Israeli government believed it could negotiate with Hamas to keep a ceasefire; Israel did *not* believe Hamas's "word": its charter to destroy Jews and the Jewish State; Israel "permitted" Qatar to fund Hamas. But Hamas et al. will follow Muhammed in his "deal" with the Jewish community to not attack them; then to wait until he built strength, attack and kill the Jewish community, except for the teenage daughter of the leader and "marry" her. This "sin"—not believing the genocidal aims of destroying Jews—hopefully has passed: *believe* Hamas/Qatar/Iran that they want Jews destroyed. Believe them.

One other near-"sin." We (at least the West) didn't fully believe the words, the repeated statements by mortal enemies of Jewish Israel

Let us be clear on this. These are not "sins" committed by the murdered. But there are unconscious self-defeating failings that we can recognize and repair.

I ask that you accompany me on this "voyage" even though unlike Danté I do not have the singing "terza rhyme" of Danté's musical language. And you can choose not to accompany me on this arduous, painful journey. You can choose not to do so. Should you join me, you need really to *listen* to those who have been through and continue to go through the experiences of Hell like those Danté met. Should you join me, see this Hell through their eyes, their senses (e.g., the stench of burnt flesh), their words, their memories.

Recall that none of our three heroes is tested hellishly. Rather, they go through as the only living beings who traverse the dead and learn from their suffering. We cannot; we don't presume to fully "understand" their suffering. Those who have been truly traumatized (a word overused in America); as many post-traumatic stress disorder (PTSD) true suffers will tell us: "you can't understand." We can only listen to the witnesses, as Elie Wiesel implored us. Listen.

We, like Odysseus, Aeneas, and Danté may benefit, learn our roles in the future. Recall the outcomes of our three Antique Hell voyagers.

Odysseus's future is to return to his wife, his son, and resume ruling his kingdom, which has fallen into disarray.

For Aeneas, it is to remarry, to build Rome into a nation that will rule wisely over others.

For Danté, it is to gain wisdom, feel absolved of his sins to reach Paradisical Beatrice, the love of his life.

I have some experience as a listener to witnesses from Hells, both father and mother. I have been until now too reluctant to recount their stories; these are their stories and I wish to be judged by my own achievements. But it is time now to recount even briefly, my "training."

Bellow's one-eyed Professor Sammler remarks that he doesn't consider himself as surviving the Shoah; he and others like him, only "lasted." Lasting is not surviving. Even surviving is barely enough. As Sammler recounts in his Upper West Side room, he barely lives. But he sees both his heart and the world around him clear-eyed.

Lasting is not living. Our task is to help those who have lasted through October 7 to reestablish life.

"*Sammler*" is Yiddish for "collector." And a collector he is—of observations, of what he sees with his remaining eye, the other one blinded by an SS man's strike. Sammler collects observations that complement his memories of good (the Oxford-trained Polish journalist who interviewed HG Wells) and of evil (buried alive with his murdered wife and hundreds of others by the SS and Polish helpers) and of the mundanities of Manhattan in the late 1900s, as it borders on incivility. (We see this Manhattan today on Columbia's campus and the administration's inability to maintain safety for Jews, even civility.) We listen to his memory-infused witnessing. And, as we will hear from Bettelheim (1979), "collecting," like "surviving," like "lasting" are not the same as integrating.

My training as a listener—for what you will hear in this chapter are stories after October 7 from those who survived—my training began in childhood. How was I "qualified" to be as King Solomon pleaded to God, to have a *lev shomeah*, a hearing heart?[2] My father, born and raised in Lodz in a middle-class family, was orphaned at eight when his father died after a progressive illness. My father, astute at math, was accepted at the Warsaw Polytechnic Institute (when Jews were quota-ed), but with the arrival of the Nazis, he did his "studies" in several Labor Concentration Camps, until the Warsaw Ghetto fell, then through a procession of Concentration Camps, until he was "graduated" to Auschwitz.

He recalls his introduction to Mengele. My father, having been kicked in the head, had wound paper on his wound to stave the blood. He noticed who got waved to the right (as I recall)—elderly, children—and who to the left—the physically able. When Mengele waved him to the right, my father tore off the ersatz bandaid and dove into the pack of the living.

Most of his stories he told with little emotion, just the facts. Much of it came when I was eight, my sister nine, and my mother in the hospital having given birth to my baby sister. In some way that I now forget, my sister and I asked him about Camp ("Kemp," he pronounced it, in a clipped manner). He gathered us to the corner of the kitchen, a niche by the back door and sat down on the low trash can, the kind with a chrome convex metal lid and foot pedal. He sat us on his lap and he spoke.

Once in the icy winter, to make an experiment, the SS commanded all the men to line up to watch a test, very scientific. The SS took a Jew and plunged him headfirst into a large metal oil barrel filled with water. The surface was frozen, so they had to break the ice with his head. Then they watched to see how long it would take for the man to stop kicking, to drown. As a boy, in my mind's eye I saw—I return to "our minds' eyes" later—I saw the man's stiff legs as if knees were frozen straight, click-clacking against the metal rim. More likely, the man desperately thrashed about.

Advice from my father. The bunks were four high. Most men, too exhausted, took the lower bunks. He took the highest. Why? At night they would delouse. Drop the lice. Take the highest bunk.

Advice from my father. When you get the piece of bread, eat it all right away. ("But, *Tatte*, I read someplace, maybe Viktor Frankl, that you should hide a piece in the bed straw for later.") No. It will be stolen.

Advice from my father. A longer dissertation on "How I got more soup." First, the German night guard, who said he had a son my age at home, made a deal. I should wash the floors on my knees at night. He would nap on the steps outside. He gave me a bolt. If I see his commander coming to check, I should chuck the bolt to wake the guard. He trusted me. Then, as a reward, he got me to ladle out the soup. Why that's good? If you ladle, you get the last soup on the bottom, more solids. And sometimes even two bowls left, which I shared. That's how to get more soup.

Practical advice he gave me.

In the coal mines was a conveyor belt to move the huge coal chunks up. Some men were too exhausted to walk out of the mine, so they crouched on the conveyer between the chunks. But sometimes the chunks shifted, crushed them. Always walk out of the mine. We had coal delivered through a chute into the basement: I saw them with new eyes after such stories. And the fierce fire in the belly of our furnace meant Auschwitz chimneys. The dead birds at the base of our chimney for me were the Jews who were sent up the chimneys as ash and smoke.

Near the end of the war, many German mechanics were moved to the Russian front. The SS needed men to repair their cars—Mercedes, of course, but also pre-War Cadillacs, which they treasured. One morning at roll call, an SS holds up a micrometer and asks, "What's this?" Now, I know that sometimes when you answer, they answer with a bullet to the head. But I answer, "micrometer" and I get moved from the coal mines to maintaining cars.

The first day, an SS tells me to wash his car. So I did. When I'm done, he puts on a white glove. Wipes it *under* the running board and shows me dirt. Beats me. Next time I clean under the running board.

"How did you survive?" I asked.
"Where there's life, there's hope."
One day, an SS takes to kicking my father's younger brother in the belly. Over and over. Even when the boy was down. My father held him in the bunk all night as his brother writhed to death. In the morning, he asked to bury his brother. The SS looked at him dismissively.
On another occasion, next to a deep ditch they had dug, an SS took to kicking my father down the ditch. My father crawled out and the SS kicks him down. My father recalls the *Shtivelen*, the black polished, shiny calf-high boots. He's kicked again and again as he crawls out. Then the SS leaves. My father's compatriots load him into a wheelbarrow to carry him back to the camp entrance. But, as they approach, my father knows that if he's wheeled in, he will likely be taken to the "infirmary" from which most leave feet first, dead. So he crawled out and walked into the camp.
I should learn from this advice.
When we move into the first house we have ever owned, some seven years into emigration, it has a gas fireplace in the dining room. My father disconnects it and blocks the gas line. "Why?" I ask. "Enough gas in Auschwitz."
I ask if we could have a chain-link fence around our yard like the other neighbors. These were fun to climb over and venture between the garages. I even get pointy shoes, then called, insensitively, Puerto Rican fence climbers. He: "I had enough fences in my life."
Bruno Bettelheim remarked that many read or know of Anne Frank's *Diary*, the writings of a murdered Jewish girl. But no one reads Margo Minco's *Bitter Herbs*; likely you haven't heard of it. This is the story of a Dutch girl *who survived* because her father trained and trained (and trained again) his daughter: if there is a knock at the door, the father will answer, he will delay the SS while the daughter and mother should jump out the back window and hide in the special ditch he had dug beneath shrubs. And not come out. No matter what they heard. Yet, as Dara Horn (2022) writes in her compelling, thoughtful book, people like dead Jews, and stories about dead Jews. Living Jews are anathema. Especially strong, living Jews. Jews even frustrated the historian Otto Spengler, whose treasured hypothesis is that every civilization rises, contributes to mankind, and then collapses on itself. And the damn Jews, per Spengler, just won't disappear, won't fall. Although many have tried to destroy them, Jews get knocked down; just won't *stay* down.

Let's return to my teacher, Bettelheim, who did his time in Birkenau Concentration Camp, although it was just before the gas chambers. His book *Surviving* looks critically at what it means to "survive" and what remains intact or can be rebuilt. The section, provocatively titled "Unconscious Contributions to One's Undoing," begins with an honest look at *our* reactions to Anne Frank's diary, continues with a hard look at Hannah Arendt's *Eichmann in Jerusalem* (and our reactions to it), and settles in with "Surviving," which takes a harsh, critical gaze on Wertmüller's *Seven Beauties*, movie, a visual essay on the Camps and *how we react* to this. This essay was some 30 years after the Shoah was brought to "rest" by Allied victories. And I emphasize, it was the United States, along with variable allies (the closest were the British, next, incompetently so, the French, and by default, the Soviets, or really Stalin). No Jewish State existed, the only Jews who helped bring about the collapse of the Nazi evil were those who served under other flags and the very few whose futile often tragic efforts at rebellion from within (my father among them at Warsaw).

We begin with a general principle we have learned from psychoanalysis about growth, about overcoming travail. "*integration* of a truly important experience requires both that we deal constructively *with what it did to us* as an inner experience, and also that *we do something about it* in our actions relating to it" (1979, 241; Bettelheim's italics).

Coming to terms with adverse events, such as child abuse, Bettelheim suggests, means first, being able to recount what was done to oneself, second, one's inner reactions; but to fully grasp and overcome this, why this was done to oneself. At least why we imagine this was done to us. For instance, my writing in this chapter is an attempt to master my subjective reactions to October 7th. This means not only recounting what happened in the towns bordering Gaza, not only recounting what I hear from others who survived or even who were physicians in the Soroka ER[3] of Beersheva, but also, and especially, why I have and am reacting the way I do to these experiences. Including how it evokes stories from my father. Mastery means not only intellectual recounting but integrative work—integrating emotional reactions with cognitive efforts, the "marriage" of Psyche (the rational) with Eros (the passion). This will mean, at times, recognizing uncomfortable, inconvenient feelings and thoughts. Why do I feel guilt? Why did I survive? How did I "contribute" to this horror, such as by *not* living in Israel, but rather, enjoying the fleshpots of America?

Let's turn to *Anne Frank*. More specifically *our* reactions to her diary.

Three kinds of reactions, Bettelheim argues, deal with the horrors of the camps, and for this chapter, October 7.

1. A form of denying it happened: that only a small number of deranged, perverted perpetrators did these horrific acts. But, today, the GoPro self-filming by Hamas itself should[4] defeat this argument. One would think.

2. Deny the acts altogether by calling it propaganda (as do some Palestin-ian/Hamas supporters, even claiming that Israelis staged these horrors—despite GoPro Hamas evidence);
3. Repress the evidence quickly. For instance, the young woman survivor of the Nova festival who tattooed on her arm: "We will dance again."

We can learn from our reactions to *Anne Frank* versus ours (and others' reactions to October 7; contrast and compare). For instance, with modern media, we can literally *see* what happened on October 7 and thereaf-ter; we learn more quickly (but also can be distorted via AI and other means) what has happened. On the other hand, like with Hitler, many did not believe his word, Hitler's promise from his early *Mein Kampf* through the 1930s and into the actions of the Camps: that he was determined to exterminate (a word used for vermin) the Jews. So too, it appears as if the world won't believe the clear and firm words of Hamas/Hezbollah/Iran (and many Imams) that the Jews should be exterminated. Hitler meant it; they mean it.

Bettelheim carefully does not take issue with the girl, the gentle Anne Frank, her moving and humane story of her tender, thoughtful development. Rather he looks at *our* reactions to this story and with greater difficulty the probably unconscious contributions to the Frank family's destruction from the father and many more Jews like him. Recall that Mr. Frank found a hiding place with no exit and then tried to carry on life as before, teaching the clas-sics to his children, even taking in another family, all the while relying on the neighbors not to squeal. In contrast, we read about other families who real-ized they could not survive together and chose to separate. Minco's is but one example (1957). My Yiddish literature teacher in high school, Dr. Chamaides, who was a pediatric cardiologist, was sent by his Polish father, a rabbi, to live in a Catholic Church when he was a boy. His family was incinerated. He survived, kept his Yiddish identity, and also married a Catholic. Yehuda Nir's painful *The Lost Childhood*, a memoir of a nine-year-old's survival—his own—is another, this mother divvying up Yehuda and his sister and herself after the father is murdered by the SS.

When the Germans overran Poland, my mother's mother told her, the eld-est, to take one sister (of five siblings) and escape to Russia. My grandmother and grandfather and others remained behind; all were killed by the Nazis, save my Uncle Avram, who survived, barely. When the 15-year-old Avram was told to bury the Jews shot in a mass grave, some still writhing, he refused. The SS grabbed my uncle's shovel, smacked him in the forehead, and my uncle began digging. Years later, I noticed as a child that my uncle had a large "Y"-shaped vein that bloomed on his forehead into his bald pate as he shouted (which was often); I thought that this was the remnants of that SS's shovel. His shouting, I also thought, was a remnant of the Camps. Avram's is one kind of "survival." But my grandmother seemed to know that the family would not survive staying together.

My father, living in middle-class Lodz, sleeping with three brothers in a bed[5] recalls his widowed mother inviting German Jewish refugees to stay with them as did other Jews in Lodz. Some of the German Jews, looking around their Polish hosts' digs, complained that they smelled bad, looked dirty, these homes of hosts . . . and returned to Germany, most likely perishing in the (not so clean) Camps.

Staying together as a family was the hardest way to go underground (Bettelheim, 248). And Mr. Frank could have armed himself, although this might not have saved the entire family. My father recalls that he was chosen in the Warsaw Ghetto to run guns and ammunition since he was blond and blue-eyed. He did say that the guns bought from the Poles were often rusted and the ammunition didn't match the guns. But they were *doing* something.

Bettelheim's point is *not to criticize* the Franks but *to hold us, us, accountable* for how *we* romanticize, even admire their manner of not coping. *Hold us accountable* for our unconscious selves. Even our reactions to the (fictionalized) last words of Anne Frank's book raise questions about us readers; "In spite of everything, I still believe that people are really good at heart." Really? We should believe this fictionalized ending? As Bettelheim says,

This improbable sentiment is supposedly from a girl who had been starved to death . . . watched her sister meet the same fate . . . knew that her mother had been murdered . . . watched untold thousands of adults and children being killed.

Words are not justified by her diary. Yet many readers find these words like an emollient, as if to deny the horror that man can do to man. We have not heard, and hopefully will not hear, such silly fictional words attributed to the survivors of October 7. In fact, one former peacenik farmer who survived and had worked toward coexistence with his Gazan neighbors now admits that the only thing he wants to see between his farm and the Sea is potato fields, just potato fields.

We are not here to blame survivors. Not those murdered. Rather, let us explore the loss of mature emotional and cognitive mechanisms.

Submission to . . . the Nazi state (or any totalitarian state . . .) often led both to the disintegration of . . . well-integrated personalities and to a return to an immature disregard for the dangers of reality.

Reading external reality accurately takes relatively intact inner reality, and one can't act with good self-preservation if one can't read external reality accurately.

In a later essay, Bettelheim points out that the danger facing modern society lies in the remarkable power of totalitarian states, *including* its almost magnetic attraction to some in democratic societies (e.g., Tucker Carlson's marvels over Soviet groceries or subways running on time). A Midwest

American journalist I met in Jerusalem sang praises over his previous posting in Damascus (before the horrendous slaughter and gassing of its citizens by Assad, crossing Obama's "red line"): compared to Jerusalem, Damascus was so clean, so civilized. So much for his journalistic objectivity. But then, his current apartment was over the Arab bus station near the Damascus gate, the Arab bus fleets' gassy smoke belching over his paltry, spindly vegetable garden. He was excited to return to Kansas with his Syrian fiancé, who later dumped him once she got US citizenship.

What we will hear from contemporary Israelis is the disintegration of previously well-integrated personalities. A well-regarded psychiatrist now suffers from insomnia, hypervigilance, sudden high blood pressure, and is unable to permit himself to attend the theater or walk through a flowered field. He has borderline diabetes now. When he hears the Hospital helicopter descend almost daily even today, he trembles, as he knows it will bear the broken bodies of Israeli soldiers from Gaza. He works with frightened families—secular Jews, Bedouin, Orthodox Jews—then, his mind is derailed by a text message from his sons that they are being deployed to either the "North" or Gaza. You've heard his poignant plaint: how can he work as a psychiatrist when his mind is at the front with his sons?

Denial. I overhear in whispered but fierce Hebrew a debate between our usually laid-back bodyguard and our somewhat *laissez-faire* tour guide over some tourists wish a late-night stroll from the Western Wall to the restaurant in the Old City. Ro'i ("my shepherd," in translation) says, "It's too dangerous in the winding alleys of the Old City; knife attacks; a rolled grenade." E., our scholarly guide, responds, "But it's a short distance, maybe ten minutes." Ro'i counters, "If you let them do this, I cannot protect them. The decision and outcome will be on you." And E. accedes. Denial of danger by both the naive tourists and the knowledgeable tour guide. Ro'i, I know, discreetly packs a pistol. When my children were fearful of my trip in December to Israel, I mentioned this to Ro'i. He said. "I will FaceTime them." He did so and said something like this. "Your father the doctor will sit near me. I am his shepherd. I will protect him. I will send him home well." My boys were overjoyed.

Denial, a first step toward permitting one's destruction with the SS. Lengyel (1947), who successfully escaped the gas chamber selection, describes fellow prisoners who denied knowing about the crematoria within a few yards. Her fellow prisoners even reported to their "supervisors" that Lengyel was escaping. Bettelheim points out that when the prisoners give up the will to live (the extreme case is the *Musselman*), they are "in the thrall of the murdering SS not only physically but also psychologically" (p. 256). While physical survival was for the most part in the hands of the SS and their minions (often gleeful sadistic Polish, Ukrainian, and Czechs), to some degree, and only to some degree, psychological survival was still possible. But *how* do we permit ourselves to learn, to listening to our unconscious wishes and thoughts, *including those that may be self-destructive*, at the hands of the manipulative death drive?

"When the world goes to pieces and inhumanity reigns supreme . . . one must radically reevaluate all of what one has done . . . in order to know how to act" (Bettelheim, p. 257). This means going beyond physical survival. Bellow in his Mr. Sammler describes the empty shell, like some katydid encrusted on a tree trunk, as "survival"; Wiesel and Primo Levy describe how much one must work to maintain one's humanity in the face of inhumanity and afterward. Integrate both emotional reactions and thoughts. This is what the fictionalized Odysseus, Aeneus, and Danté learned: integrating what they have seen, the horrors, *the horrors*, of Hell, then taking this as they return to a higher life.

I realize that this interlude earlier, these allusions to Bettelheim and Wiesel and Primo Levi (2015), is a way to soften our descent. But descend we must into the Hell of October 7, not to gaze, like voyeurs, not just to feel grateful that we were not attacked but to learn from those who suffered, some dead, some alive.

A caution. What is seen is not unseen. Even though these are words, even though I describe what was described to me, like Danté's poetic accounts, the words will inscribe themselves into our visual, or corporal, our sensate being. By inscribe, I mean like Kafka's *The Penal Colony* (2000), where a man's "sins" are carved into his skin. Caution to those who enter. We will not quote Danté's "Lasciate Esperanza, voi ch'intraté. 'Abandon all hope those who enter here'": without hope, no future.

The Hamas broadcast with glee video of the horrors they did to humans. I recount what I wrote at the chapter's beginning. A woman is raped from behind as another terrorist cuts off her breast, tossing it about before discarding it. Then she is shot in the head. Babies are thrown live into ovens before their parents. A parent is bound back to back to its child and both are shot dead. A woman murdered dead found with nails driven into her vagina. Men dead, with genitals shot off. Faces blown away. A woman found dead with her pelvis pulverized from multiple rapes. Children found dead in a shelter after being grenaded. A young boy survives with belly wounds because his 16-year-old brother jumps on him and takes bullets. From Kibbutz Be'eri are four graves—shoulder to shoulder—of the Even family—father, mother, and two sons. One son remains alive because his teenage brother also jumped on his body to take the bullets. A Hamas terrorist films a young boy—perhaps six—whose eyes have been gouged out by Hamas; the boy is telling his older brother that he cannot see and that their father is dead; a terrorist calmly combs their fridge for a Coke to guzzle during this. A teen, knowing that he is dying, asks his parents that he buried with his surfboard. They are all killed. There is more, more too much more. I write this with tears in my eyes and heart. I do not want my children to read this.

The number of dead, some 1,200, doesn't even tell us enough. Kidnapping is almost an afterthought; those kidnapped, raped, tortured, murdered. Enough, enough. This goes beyond Danté's Hell, for it is done on earth by those who have the *appearance* of human beings.

And since then, demonstrators at Columbia University regale over October 7 (including faculty members) call for more October 7th. A Hamas leader *promises* that there will be more. Jewish students at American Universities fear for their own safety; a Barnard rabbi advises students to leave campus as the University cannot protect them. University presidents equivocate on protecting Jewish students. Jewish students are given "permission" to complete studies by Zoom; at Yale, Jewish-appearing students are barred from campus by protestors. But all the latter in this paragraph palls in the face of what was done on October 7; what Iran's mullahs intended on April 13, 2024—170 drones, 120 surface-to-surface ballistic missiles, and 30 cruise missiles, destruction measured in tons—the wipeout of Jews.

There is historical precedence. In the 1929 Arab riot and murder of Jews, the Arabs also sliced off women's breasts, as if murder was not sufficient. We could go further back in time, as historians of warfare can, to find comparable brutality. But this may be enough for now. This abominable hatred and murder and torture is not new but not expected in the Jewish State. This, the State must rectify; psychological treatment takes place, as Winnicott said of British children during the Nazi "V"-bombings, after the military protects our safety. And, as the United States and Allies did with Germany and Japan, they must completely vanquish the enemy.

But what can we do for the living? Listening and doing. These are our two tasks to repair those who have been subjected to such horrors and those affected by the echo of these horrors, including some readers. How can we do these so that we, like Odysseus/Aeneus/Danté emerge more whole from Hell?

This we begin to answer here, but expect that our answers will be revised, strengthened by those to whom we listen, including to those who read this.

Listening is a form of witnessing. Jonathan Shay, a remarkable psychiatrist/neurologist who worked with Veteran's Administration soldiers with PTSD, gives a key. Sit with groups of soldiers; let them speak with each other. Watch as they begin to hear, really hear, what their colleagues have gone through and together find ways to emerge from their tunnel-visioned darkness. For acute stress disorder (ASD) with soldiers at the North African front in WWII, Grinker and Spiegel discovered a specific way of listening and watching. They initiated the principles of proximity, immediacy, and expectation of recovery (later labeled by Solomon (2008) with Lebanese war soldiers as P.I.E.). Prior to Grinker, soldiers who succumbed to ASD were sent back from the front, eventually home to the US, a trip that could take months. By that time, ASD converted to chronic PTSD, at times, life-long disabling. Instead, Grinker treated soldiers with ASD near the front. He used an intravenous barbiturate drug, given slowly to induce a slight somnolence yet awareness. Then, he asked open-ended questions about what happened. Many soldiers who otherwise could not "remember" or articulate the events that led to acute stress, would not only speak, but often leap from the bed, crouch to the floor holding their (imaginary) rifle, and reenact the events that traumatized them. Subsequent sessions often worked without the barbiturate. Then, Grinker returned them to the front with their units.

Others (Solomon, 2008) since then have shown that immediate and proximal treatment (close to time and place of trauma) was most effective. And returning at least soldiers—and we will argue, also children—to their normal peer groups helps.

We speak of war research with soldiers, as this is the area where post-trauma work has been most extensive and most effectively studied. We will extend this to children and families: treat the children close in time, close in proximity (once that proximity is physically safe), and expect that they will respond well to thoughtful treatment.

Another gem from Grinker's *Men Under Stress* (1945) is that the "clinical picture" of ASD may vary widely: some soldiers present as psychotic, others with lesser symptoms. It matters less the overt presentation; the treatment principles remain the same: *treat soon; treat near; return to the "unit."*

The power of one's peer group was demonstrated, ironically, in a study of WWII German soldiers by Janowitz (1960) a Jewish sociologist at the University of Chicago. While in the US army, after the Allies' victory, he asked: why is it that German soldiers continued to fight so hard when they knew that the German army was losing the war? His answer (from the soldiers) was *not* for the Fatherland, *not* for Hitler. Rather out of camaraderie with fellow soldiers in one's unit. An Israeli soldier who was in the very elite *Shayetet* (Navy Seals) taught me this. I was introduced to Moishek as one of the bravest soldiers in the 1956 assault at the treacherous Mitla Pass, *a hero, others called him*. But, when we sat together at his Kibbutz's cafeteria after picking avocados that morning while drinking muddied *Botz* coffee oversweetened in thick-handled porcelain mugs, Moishek turned to me. "Why did I run into bullets? Why? I looked to my right, I looked to my left and I saw my buddies running into bullets. I couldn't stop. I had to run *with* them. I'm no hero." Yes, we can ascribe some of this to his kibbutznik modesty. But we can also believe him, especially for a kibbutznik raised with multiple non-sibling "siblings." He has a feel for fighting with his soldier siblings that he will fight with them, even for them (Szajnberg, 2006; Szajnberg, 2013).

Another example of connection with one's unit (and leadership) is more recent. "Ro'i" (I call him "My Shepherd" here) is a leader (also an officer) in one of the elite soldier units, in this case Golani. Once, long ago, Golani soldiers were considered "gorillas," that is, knuckle dragging not so smart tough guys; today, they are both smart and tough. After October 7, as Ro'i was about to lead his unit across the line into Gaza, he—of few words—gave some directions of how the unit was to move, targets, dangers. Then, he paused. He looked back at the remnants of a town that had been attacked by the Hamas murderers but not wiped out. He nodded with his head to the lights in the homes. He then said, in a last whisper, "Look, look. For *this* you fight." This creates group cohesion.

Yet one more example from a soldier returning from West Bank soldiering, a member of *Duvdevan* ("cherry"), a unit whose job description is something like this: be fluent in Palestinian Arabic, preferably "look" Arab, dress Arab, sit in West Bank cafés maybe playing *Shesh Besh* (backgammon). Listen to gossip. Listen for planned terrorist attacks against civilians. Then, at night, with your unit, go into the town, approach the house of the suspected terrorist, and arrest him. Now, I asked this member of "*Duvdevan*," why he fought so hard and why in such a dangerous unit. This father of four, this architect (I disguise the details) answered. "If they kill me, next they will kill my wife, then my children." That was his simple answer. A different motivation than group cohesion. Or a different group: his family. I knew that his home was but some two kilometers from Tulquarm, a West Bank hive of suicide bombers.

Colonel John Spencer has summarized the importance of group cohesion and its "ingredients" in his monumental *Connected Soldiers: Life, Leadership, and Social Connections*. A soldier and officer for several decades in the elite Rangers unit, he now teaches modern urban warfare at West Point. While too lengthy for here, I touch on his major points. Combat effectiveness depends on three factors: (1) Interests (survival, normative, pay, etc.), (2) motivation (moral, group cohesion), and (3) military (discipline, tactical, administrative, organizational command system) as found in Napoleon's command (Spencer, 2022).

But a major factor for why soldiers fight is group cohesion, both task and social cohesions (Stouffer et al., 1949).[6] Even as late as the (now questionable) Iraq war, cohesion was an important factor (Wong et al., 2003).[7]

Why do I write so much about military cohesion? For two reasons.

First, the military is one of mankind's oldest enduring (Western) institutional organizations, and the second is the Catholic Church. We can learn much from its robust management of groups of people and how to effectively manage morale. For, morale among survivors of October 7 and its aftermath(s)—morale/anxiety of the parents which will affect the children—is a primary ingredient. Anna Freud and colleagues demonstrated how children's response to the V-Bombing of London was dependent significantly on the mothers' reactions (Freud and Burlingame, 1949).[8]

Second, Israel, as one of its retired generals remarked to me (Szajnberg, 2006), is a *militarized*, but *not militant* nation. Most of its citizens serve in the military and perhaps because of this, most *do not want their* children to go to war. To flip a phrase from Golda Meier, Israelis love their children more than they dislike Arabs who hate them. Hence, what we learn from military cohesion and organization may make sense to Israelis, particularly parents.

———

I ask that you join me as witnesses on this infernal journey.

Witnessing? What is this witnessing we are trying to achieve? Remember King Solomon. At the start of Solomon's reign, God appears in his dream and says, "Ask. What shall I give you?"

Solomon requests to be granted a "hearing heart."

And God's "interpretation" (which could be a decent psychoanalytic one) is that Solomon desires "to discern and understand justice" (3:11). We look forward to model Solomon's life and integrate, discern, and understand justice transforming it into "wisdom." Solomon is known for his wisdom. (He is also known for his middle name, Yadidiah, literally "hand in hand," figuratively, "(God's) good friend.") We need to develop *hearing hearts* and possibly achieve wisdom.

There are a least *six levels of witnessing*.

First, those who *went through* the horrors of the Nova festival or their kibbutzim/towns ravaged.

Second, those who *have seen* the broken bodies, charred babies in ovens, limbs chopped off, and beheaded torsos. A psychologist for the *Shayetet* (Navy Seals) unit meets with them after each major action. *Shayetet* are trained to kill (and face their own deaths). When they were called up on October 7, one unit stopped a second wave of Hamas terrorists invading from the Mediterranean onto Israel proper. Killed them all. Every one. Yet the *Shayetet* men tell me that all their experiences did not prepare them for what they saw in Be'eri and surrounding towns. For, their first task before being deployed to stop invaders, *their first task* was to gather the bodies of slaughtered Jews. These young men (in their twenties) were not prepared for the horrifying scenes I only sketch earlier. This was seared into their eyes at Be'eri. For Be'eri, these men sought help, treatment.

The Israeli army, unfortunately, has had much experience with treating the impact of horrors, true trauma, on soldiers. We will continue to learn from them.

Third, we have the civilians, including children who were *kidnapped*, some of whom were rescued. For these, we are hearing; the Israeli government and psychiatric services are providing succor. For the children especially, this will be a challenge, particularly if family members were killed, often before their eyes.

Fourth, we are left with groups who *went and continue to go through attempted annihilations* of October 7, the not-so-small Hells of continued bombings, such as Iran's attempts on April 13, or Hezbollah/Yemen/Hamas rockets continuing.

Fifth, we have the psychiatrists and colleagues who we expect to treat those traumatized *and* somehow overcome their own vicissitudes to be available to treat others. One resident psychiatrist began by telling me that her father was murdered on October 7.

We must sketch out the beginning ascent from Hell. How do we achieve the wisdom that our triumvirate of "heroes" achieved to build better lives?

Sixth, us. We are, you readers and this voyager, listening to the previous experiences, witnessing the profound impact of living through Hell. How are we affected? This I leave for the reader to recognize. We are in good company; we are like those who read Danté, listen to Virgil, and draw our conclusions about suffering and Hell. And, most importantly, we should emerge with some wisdom gleaned from the sufferers who speak to us. We are like startled Danté, when Cavalcanté erupts erect from his flaming tomb when he hears Danté's familiar Tuscan accent. Cavalcanté poignantly wants to know, to learn "Does my son still live?" only to collapse in his burning tomb. We can ask over the course of this journey "(How) do the survivors still live?"

But before getting to specifics, I will quote from a letter by Naftali Bennett, former elite Maglan soldier, former Prime Minister, that he read to his family about Pesach. In it, he addresses a major ailment in Israeli society that has weakened it over the past two years, an ailment in society that is closest to a "sin" that is an inner weakness. As Bennett tills the soil, he identifies and uproots the weeds and roots or discord of the past two years, which will impede planting the seeds and seedlings of repair. This "sin" we can overcome as part of emerging from Hell. Recall that the fine Danté was hampered from ascending to Paradise by the three frightful beasts that represented his sins. His tour through Hell helped him overcome these "sins." We too can overcome at least this one "sin," the *Sinat Chinam* free-floating anger at brothers and sisters that jeopardized and jeopardizes Israel. This made Israel look vulnerable to its enemies. For, Israel's truest enemies are like hyenas—looking for weak prey to devour, tear apart[9]—children, elderly, women, citizens—no armed combatants for these cowardly hyenas.

Earlier, I summarized Spencer's ideas about cohesion in the army. He describes two types: task cohesion and social cohesion. The first, task cohesion, is some agreement, consensus of the future task at hand—to overtake a hill, to jump and parachute out of a plane at under 1,000 feet, to cover your teammates. The second, social cohesion, is a sense of connectedness with the team at hand. In general, we have learned from Roman army times until today, a small team needs some 8–15 members to be effective. Less than eight, one achieves less (except for rare special ops); over 15, and a leader has trouble staying in touch with all members of the team out in the field. And staying in touch (a term I prefer to the colder, "communication") is a necessary ingredient for team efficacy and leadership.

I review this to turn to the cohesion of Israeli society after October 7. Prior to that, some tens of thousands of Israelis were protesting, blocking traffic, harassing the prime minister on vacation, and so on, in opposition to the (majority-elected)[10] government's decisions. I do not take a position on who was right or wrong. I only emphasize that this opposite of cohesion, this intra-societal conflict, jeopardized the Jewish State. The animosity was tangible, the faces contorted with hate. Projection—that psychic process of taking our innermost negative traits and splashing them onto another—prevailed: the other side is all bad, wrong, and even evil. Both task cohesion and social cohesion are jeopardized. Fortunately, tragically, task cohesion—the task of surviving as a Jewish people and State—remains robust. But October 7th had to provoke this transformation.

I recall during the Second Lebanese War, one of my soldiers (I often say "my" soldiers, as I became close with them) returned drained from Lebanon.[11] He described confusing orders emanating from Tel Aviv command to his unit in Lebanon—move from this house to that house, then back to this house, then don't move, and then move. But he said, referring to the Jewish people trying to live along the Lebanese front (the *Oref*, or "neck") and to his fellow soldiers, he said, "The Jewish people are strong."

Bear with me as I quote extensively from Naftali Bennett's words to his family for Pesach. I do this without endorsing Bennett the former prime minister. I endorse his diagnosis of the societal ailment of Israel and its repair.

Bennett begins with the dark quote from Ezekiel, that hallucinatory prophet. I begin with words from God to Moses to be intoned to the children of Israel's (our) ears in *Dvarim* (Deuteronomy) 30:19.

הַעִדֹתִי בָכֶם הַיּוֹם אֶת־הַשָּׁמַיִם וְאֶת־הָאָרֶץ הַחַיִּים וְהַמָּוֶת נָתַתִּי לְפָנֶיךָ הַבְּרָכָה וְהַקְּלָלָה וּבָחַרְתָּ בַּחַיִּים לְמַעַן תִּחְיֶה אַתָּה וְזַרְעֶךָ:

"I witness before you today the sky and the earth, the life and the death, I gave before you blessing and curse; and **choose life** to live and for your seed."

Choose Life.

Bennett begins with Ezekiel, that strident prophet:

"וָאֶעֱבֹר עָלַיִךְ וָאֶרְאֵךְ מִתְבּוֹסֶסֶת בְּדָמָיִךְ"

"וָאֹמַר לָךְ בְּדָמַיִךְ חֲיִי"

"And I passed over you and saw you wallowing in your blood, and I said to you, 'In your blood live' and I said to you In your blood live!"

Ezekiel finishes with "I rinsed the blood from you and rubbed you with oil."

Ezekiel says only to "live." Yet, on Pesach, Bennet points out, we are accustomed to saying "*hag sameach,*" *happy* holiday.

His children demand of their father, "*Abba.*" How can we say "happy" after October 7? Or "How can we say 'freedom' when so many are still hostages?" And we might add, many more feel held psychologically hostage by Hamas.[12] We will hear from them in our last chapter.

The Passover *seder* truly begins with the four children's questions. The previous questions are simple, yet powerful.

Here is how Bennett tries to answer these questions of "happy,'" or of freedom. These inform our hearts today. I translate and edit slightly.[13]

This year we are not happy. Happy is an action instruction towards ourselves:

Don't stew in the depression of the difficult situation. Take initiative, **unite, work together to get us out of the dark pit we have fallen into and into rebuilding the State of Israel.** (My emphasis)

The Haggadah calls us to come out of slavery to freedom . . ., from mourning . . . from darkness to great light, from slavery to redemption.

. . .**be active** . . . leave . . . disasters of death and helplessness; **act to** create, freedom and sovereignty.

3,300 years ago, from a terrible unbearable slavery . . . (by) Egyptians (who) murdered our baby boys, we stood up boldly: renounced our Egyptian master, crossed the Red Sea, received the Torah, united, conquered our land and established our Jewish state in the Land of Israel.

. . .76 years ago, from the abyss of the darkness of the Holocaust, we stood up,. . . united and within only three years we boldly established a Jewish state in the Land of Israel . . .

> Now our generation must act again:
> Rise from shock and depression.
> . . . unite and **re-establish** the State of Israel, (a physical state, but also a
>   state of mind).[14]
> Be strong against *external* enemies,
> Be bold *internally*:
> Break away from . . . destructive "camps":
> "The Right," "The Left," "The Religious," "The Secular," "The Haredim."
> Break away from blame:. . .
> *Our true camp is Jewish-Israeli.*
> *They* are our brothers and sisters . . . not our enemies.
> Unity does not mean be nicer;
> Unity is a condition for our existence.
> This year . . .**we tore ourselves apart from the inside;** the enemy saw this
>   and attacked us at the height of our weakness . . .
> Have courage to compromise . . .
> Unite for:
> Freedom for the kidnapped.
> Freedom from inner hatred.
> Freedom in our country."

What does this mean for our task today as psychiatrists, psychologists, mental health workers, and more so, as citizens?

We require some fertile soil of common beliefs and belief in future, a foundation upon which we can build with the specific techniques as psychiatrists.

Friends and colleagues were surprised that I "needed" (not "wanted") to go to Israel as soon as feasible after October 7; my only brief answer was, "*Kol Yisrael Arevim Zeh B'zeh.* Every Israelite is for the other." One non-Jewish good friend surprised when she learned I was going to Israel in December 2003 asked, "Do you have any family there?" My answer? "Most of my family was murdered in Europe. Their ashes cover Polish potato fields. My family is Israel." Of course, I had longer answers for those whom I knew well. When my father was in Auschwitz or my mother waiting at the Russian border with her younger sister to be admitted as refugees, there was no Jewish State and no country prepared to help them. And Jews around the world found it difficult to respond. Henry Morgenthau, Roosevelt's Secretary of Treasury, whispered into the president's ear about Jew slaughter. But Roosevelt was "deaf"; he turned back the leaky St. Louis ship, crammed with refugees nearing the US coast, and turned it back limping to Germany, where the St. Louis disgorged its Jews to the maw of murderous Nazis.

I had a certain strength of heart. Not "courage" used in the usual sense of bravery, of going into battle and such. Rather, the "courage" which comes from the French, *couer*, "heart," and in Hebrew is *ometz lev*, "strength of heart." It was strength of heart, I felt, not bravery. Not at all, bravery. My wife reminded me that I have four young children, the closest she came to suggesting I not go during active bombings from Gaza, from Hezbollah in the North, and soon, from Yemen and then Iran. But she realized that I had to go. And I did.

I suggest we leaven Bennett's Pesach talk with his children with the yeast of Bettelheim's idea of integrating heart and mind, reason and feeling. Here is another example.

On a tour through the mock-up of Khan Younis on an army base in Israel, a moonless voyage, the sergeant from reserves, perhaps 32, a father of four, a *kippat-srugah* (modern Orthodox) gives us exercises: "From where you are standing, you get incoming sniper fire from up there, that building, third floor, second window. What do you do?" We mumble, stumble in the darkness, and wait for his response. (That he would call in coordinates for rocket fire, coordinates a few yards from where he stood, over our shoulders. He trusted the pilot's accuracy.)

Then, after the tour, before we join the Maglan unit for BBQ and singing until 10:00 p.m., he tells us of his October 7. His younger brother and children are at his house for Shabbat a few minutes from the Gaza border. When his brother visits, for safety of the children, he keeps his gun and ammunition in the sergeant's room, in the bureau. At 8:00 a.m., his brother phones him—phones—"I am coming for my gun." The sergeant, still not fully awake, says "What? It's Shabbat morning, go back to bed." His brother enters, gathers his equipment, and begins to leave. The sergeant sees the look in his brother's eyes and, silently, also loads up. They drive the few minutes to Be'eri and on the road begin firing at Hamas, who have come as far as *Ofakim*. They kill terrorists, then enter *Be'eri*, to find the dead, the dismembered, the beheaded, and some alive. They load bodies, first the injured, then the dead, some 6–8 into the car, drive to safety, return for more, all the while shooting at infiltrators. Thus, they continue until about noon when they have learned about the Hamas attack. They continue for 36 hours—shooting terrorists, retrieving the living, then the dead.

We are dead silent, mouths agape, us Americans. One woman asks the "American" question, "How did you *feel* during this?"[15]

A long pause by the sergeant. Then an answer. "At those times, I do not feel, I act."

Act, like Bennett says. But it is action infused by feeling, by thought. The feeling that he recounts is not rageful anger.

Another soldier, whom I tell this tale, teaches me that there is a Hebrew saying, important for the army: "*Am boneh Tzava, boneh Am,*" "Nation builds army which builds nation." It is circular. Spencer (2022) says that every society builds its own army: different values, different cultures, different ideological systems, and build different armies. A totalitarian society (Russian, Chinese, and Nazi Germany) will build a different army than a democratic society. And a society informed by three millennia of Jewish values (and the more recent 300 years of modern democracy) builds another kind of army. The army's overall task—to defend, to attack, and to defeat—may be the same. But how the army is built, disciplined and functions, will differ.

That is, any of our recommendations or techniques for intervention, post-vention, and prevention—whatever we call it—are seeds that must be planted in the *well-prepared soil of cohesion*, both social and task oriented.

What is one cohesive task in Israel post October 7? To diminish Hamas and affiliated mortal enemies of the Jews. This is the primary task of the military, with the political as ancillary. As Clausewitz put it, "War is the continuation of policy with other means" (*On War*, 1832/1984). I remind us of Winnicott's comment earlier: when the British government asked what to do for the children in London during the V-bombing, he said to first keep them safe; the rest is (psychoanalytic) commentary.

But, to develop Bennett's call to "action," this must be guided by integration of thought and emotion, as Bettelheim said of the concentration camp experience. In a democratic society, this is the citizen's task. And in a Jewish democratic society—the Jewishness being some three millennia old, the democracy just a bit younger, born in Greece—the task of action will be infused by millennia of thoughts about how to live the good life: repair the world, be pure of heart, do not covet your neighbor's possessions (except his knowledge), do not murder, and much of the basic ten commandments elaborated by eons of commentary. We invert Cain's question to "I *am* my brother's keeper."

I remind us of the Israeli soldier returning from Lebanon II stating that the people of Israel are strong, even if the government may falter. This was echoed two decades later by a 40-year-old officer returning from Gaza. An attorney in his daily life, he volunteered for Gaza; his major role was to inform officers about the international legality of military actions. First, he said that he was shocked when he crossed into Gaza that every home and of course each school, each hospital was chock-a-block full of Hamas weapons and ammunition. Also Nazi propaganda. Recovering from that (and he repeated this several times), he looked at us flinty-eyed: Israelis are winning this war, Israelis are succeeding at tunnel discovery, destruction and both above- and belowground battles. Whatever we may hear on the news, know that the Israeli soldier knows he is winning this war. He recalls in his unit, when it came time to reserve a soldier to get a day's leave to return home, his unit's men refused to go, volunteering someone else—someone with a wife, or with children, or parents. In the end, none would take this brief leave.

His appeal to us: "Let us finish this war." The people are strong. Hopefully, the politicians will follow.

The Jewish people—a unified people, a band of brothers (and sisters) enlisted by Biblical Joseph—are the fertile ground on which we will seed our efforts for rehabilitation, for prevention, and for our children.

Hence, we leaven Bennett's call to action with the need to inform action, to inform it with an informed heart, integrating reason with emotions (Bettelheim, 1960). Just as the Psyche-Eros myth ends happily when the sensual Eros is finally wedded with the beautiful, reason-filled Psyche, so too we must calibrate and recalibrate our actions with informed hearts.

Techniques, which we generate from reason, is not sufficient if we do not integrate them with our honest emotions. And emotion needs to be sincere. Torah says do not do to others what you don't want to be done to yourself. The Christian inversion of this is to love they neighbor, do unto others what you want done to you (borrowed from Bible, Deuteronomy, *Kedoshim*). The Christian version can be infused with reaction formation—that false "goodness" that has as a force behind it of hostility. The Jewish version is more modest: don't want bad things done to you? Then don't do it to others. Less "Christian," more human. Can one truly love another as one loves oneself? Questionable without a certain falsehood behind it, from a psychoanalytic perspective. And psychoanalysts are of the skeptical sort.

Once we know we have fertile ground, which must be weeded periodically, tilled, then we can work on the specifics of how to overcome the Hell of October 7 and the continuing aftershocks of Hamas/Hezbollah/Yemen and Iran. And, like Odysseus, Aeneus, and Danté, we will be transformed by this journey through Hell. Even if we only see/hear the sufferings of its denizens, we will be changed. Our task here is to learn how to change in the direction of wisdom, in the desire and clarity of a better future.

But what are the seeds or seedlings we must plant on this prepared ground? To answer this, we can turn to the Biblical Joseph story. When Joseph assumed the mantle of leadership of his family, he implicitly decided to include all 12 brothers to build the Jewish nation, fulfilling his father's dream. Jacob on his deathbed gave specific prophecies for each son. He begins with the eldest and spices his prophecies with adversities based on the older sons' actions: Ruben, who bedded Jacob's concubine after Rachel's death, is impulsive, unstable, and will live a life accordingly. He then softens his judgments as he turns to his younger sons. Judah, who is in the middle, is also the son who beds his two sons' (widowed) wife. He will be a military leader, live by the sword. While his brothers will know that they are protected by him, the reader/listener also senses that this is a mixed blessing, to live by the sword, to be in battle.

After his father's death, Joseph's brothers fear Joseph. He reassures his brothers that he will care for them and their descendants. Further, he implicitly decides that he will include all his brothers in building a nation. After all, we might say, Joseph could have chosen only the more reliable, less impulsive, rebellious brothers to build a nation.

Moses follows Joseph's model. He leads *all* the Jews out of Egypt. Even when they complain at the Red Sea about being led out of slavery to face possible slaughter at the then-undivided Sea, he leads them all through. And, when he sends 12 spies, a "prince of each tribe" to check out the new land, only two return with promising news; the others were fearful: Joshua and

Caleb saw a land of milk and honey. The others saw inhabitants who were like giants. Moses made a strategic decision. In retrospect, he could have led only the two tribes—Caleb's and Joshua's into the land and left the rest to their own vicissitudes. Or, he could have chosen Caleb and Joshua to lead the other ten tribes and devil-take-the-hindmost. Instead, he kept all 12 together and wandered them for 40 years in the Wilderness of Zin until the slave generation died off and a new desert-hardened generation was prepared to battle to return to their land.

We face a similar analogy in contemporary Israel. There are many tribes, as Bennett says earlier. The tribes range from tiny Neturei Kartah, *charadim* of different stripes to *tzfon boni* Tel Aviniks who spend Shabbat at the beach playing *matkot*, Israeli paddle ball.

I recall a scene in Jerusalem near *Rehov Ethiopia ("Street," but more an alley)*, where I was heading to work in the child psychiatry clinic. The street— more an alley—was blocked by two groups of *charedim* each facing the other from the curbs of the narrow street. In Jerusalem, the plastic garbage bins are on wheels and the size of small Volkswagens. The *charedim* were of different tribes: one side had pants ending below the knees and socks running over three-quarter-length black pants. The other had long pants. They were battling. They had set the massive plastic bins aflame. Being plastic, the thick smoke billowed upward as if to block the sun. They would then push the bins at each other, back and forth, shouting at the other "tribe." Until the police arrive. The two tribes of *charedim* now joined in battle, turned against the police, shoving the melting, burning VW-size garbage bins at the police. *This* we can't afford.

Who is more like Reuben than Benjamin, more Judah than Issachar? In a sense we all must strive to be a Joseph, bringing our brothers and sisters into our common task: to build a people into a nation, to sustain our national sense and future.

All this is soil preparation for seedling planting.

———

Am boneh tzavah, boneh am (Nation builds army, builds nation)
Seedlings and Seeds for the future:

Bomb shelters are of two kinds in Israel. There is the *ma'amad*, with room for a family. There is the *miklat*, a communal shelter, with room for many families, which I have seen on kibbutzim or we saw—bullet-pocked, blood-stained, grenade-scorched inners—in the horrifying roadsides near the Nova festival. The pictures of the *miklatim* after October Seven, also often show paintings on the outside, evidently by trained artists of oversized sloe-eyed cats or such animals gazing out at us. Perhaps the artist was trying to portray a certain innocence, or comfort.

I recall, instead, the inside of Kibbutz Glil Yam's *miklat*. Glil Yam is an older Kibbutz located near the Mediterranean shore and now surrounded on three sides by thriving Herzliyah and the fourth side by Route 1 along the coast. This *miklat* was full of stuffies—Pooh Bear, kittens, doggies. Shlomi, who was born on this Kibbutz, told me that each stuffy was a replica of one that every child had in their home. When the children came down in that rush of "red" danger signals, they were greeted by a stuffy just like the one at home. And in the center of the ceiling of the large salon was a rotating mirrored ball, like the one from *Saturday Night Fever*. When there were no emergencies, the Kibbutz would schedule dance parties for the teens: a way of getting them acquainted with the *miklat* when there was no bombing emergency. One of the teenagers recalled going to the *miklat* when there was an emergency as a child. She thought it was a kind of party, one that last several days and nights.

The *miklat* should be decorated inside and out, but not by professional painters, rather by the children themselves. Professionals can help. For instance, after the children pick which characters they want on the walls—Mickey Mouse, Smurfs, Moomin, Rocky and Bullwinkle, even Boris and Natasha—these can be outlined by artists but painted in by the children. When Derek Miller, an adolescent psychiatrist, was recruited to Northwestern University, it built a new inpatient unit for his teens. Within days, the delinquent teens punched and kicked holes in the new drywall. Miller had an artist outline geometric designs on the repaired walls but had the teens paint in the colors. Not a single wall was marred thereafter. Involve the children in decorating these bomb-resistant refuges. And as much as feasible, favor the *miklat*, which favors and fosters community, and dilutes the idiosyncrasies of individual families, over the single family *ma'amad*, which in any case provided little security from terrorists.

Turn our children into book authors. Help them write and illustrate their own post October 7 book. And then a second book, about the future. A book about the present/past is their stories about October 7 and the bombings they continue to hear. The future book is about their hopes and dreams for what their lives will bring. With beginning, middle, and end; with past, present, and future. The advantage of the future is that we can form it, change it, express our wishes, and then learn how to manifest those wishes.

How to manifest a future? A 16-year-old girl from Ofakim recalls that Shabbat morning. The salon window was open, often the case on Shabbat. On looking out, she saw a white *tender*, a truck used by the terrorists, racing past the house. She felt something was wrong. She and the family were sheltered; only the adjacent neighborhood was attacked.

"How will you make things better for yourself?" I ask. Her answer: "Each Friday, I cook Shabbat dinner for the soldiers on the base nearby—schnitzel, felafel, humus—homemade." This is how she makes *her* life better. And when she is 18 she wants to be in the *Oketz* unit, the trained-dog unit[16] of the army. Then she will always have a "buddy" with her to fight the enemy.

After the Scud bombing of Tel Aviv by Saddam Hussein in 1991—some 42 bombs—the children were asked to draw pictures (Laor, Personal Communication). Many drew the massive, fat Scud rockets flying toward their home.

When asked how to make it funny, how to make it change for the better, the children redrew the Scuds, but now when they exploded (in the air) showering down colored balloons, or clowns, or a Scud with a painting of Saddam made a U-turn and landed on Saddam's head in Iraq. That's one way to manage a terrifying past; change it, even humorously. Let the children's imaginations with guidance, play, reverse their fears.

On my December 2023 visit to Israel, I returned to "my" Ethiopian children's school, Beit Tzipporah. It is named by Elie Wiesel after his sister who was murdered in Auschwitz. When Wiesel was looking for a charity to support in Israel, he asked for those who were most deprived, most disadvantaged. The Ethiopians, he was told. So, it was Ethiopian children he chose. And to avoid the education bureaucracy, he set up an after-school program for the children. And he paid the teachers more than the prevailing wage. The children started their after-school program with a hot meal, often the only hot meal they would have for the day. Extra meals were sent home to the parents. The classrooms were small, some 14–18 children, unlike the usual 30 or so in public classrooms. The school is in Kiryat Malachi, an old Moroccan established town north of the Negev and Ashkelon on the coast.

I worked there while I was the Freud Professor at the Hebrew University. The hour-plus commute left much time for me to reflect.[17]

I found this setting at a Shabbat lunch in Ra'anana. The Executive Director of Beit Tzipporah told me the history of the school and its connection with Wiesel. I had just finished my book on Israeli elite soldiers. I was looking for a project, something meaningful. I had heard that the Ethiopian immigrants were having more difficulties being absorbed (the Hebrew word) than previous groups. Here was a setting with children where I could learn, work, and possibly help. (As it was outside the Jerusalem Education Bureaucracy, I needed only the permission of the parents and principal.) The results of my three years at Beit Tzipporah are in my book, *Sheba and Solomon's Return: Ethiopian Children in Israel* (2013). The children's stories and pictures enlighten the book. The children's stories reveal their families, their histories, and their hope for the future. We can replicate that with our children today: the past (their history), the present, and their hoped-for futures. For each child a book. Each child. And the future book can be revised and changed and edited and made brighter with each iteration.

Here is a basic framework we can borrow from the Israeli army. The psychiatrist/psychologist consults with the officers; the officers, closer to their soldiers, transmit our suggestions. And this is not "therapy," rather it is training.[18] Training is familiar to soldiers (and education to children). A further analogy: it is best to work with officers closest to the soldier—captain, lieutenant. The colonels and generals are too far removed from the battlefield. In our analogy, if we push it, the Generals and colonels are the pedagogues in Jerusalem or the principals of schools. They are best informed by *the officers, who are the parents*.

If we follow this model, we child psychiatrists and psychologists work most directly with parents and with their approval further work with their children.

And we can work with children in a classroom (such as creating their books) or individually if a child has more acute problems. Screening instruments aid us, as we discuss later.

Now, you hear how the tone of this book shifts from Odysseus, Aeneus, and Danté, from tilling and preparing the soil of our minds and children's minds, to the nitty gritty: what can we do to help our children?

We are fortunate that since Anna Freud's (1976) pioneering work with Theresienstadt surviving children, work with war-trauma children has developed. Natti Laor in Israel has pioneered this with more contemporary Israel wars, as has Yolanda Gampel's work with Shoah descendants (1998). But Bob Pynoos and his network of colleagues (Pynoos et al., 2014) have summarized the literature and offered well-validated interviews but for brief screening and more in-depth assessment.

To be clear, Pynoos and colleagues screen for PTST, not ASD. We have a complex situation with our children; they are months away from October 7, but they continue to be under assault in war; even as I write in spring 2025, ballistic missiles are fired from Yemen. PTSD and ASD may not be easily separable. Recall the resident in psychiatry at Soroka who introduces herself by telling me her father was murdered on October 7; then I learn that she is living in temporary shelter until it is safe to move back to her home along the Gaza border. Another resident returned from outside the country with her children and her husband (beyond warrior "age") immediately dispatched himself to Gaza to fight. She and their children saw him two months later.

The four categories of PTSD symptoms will be unfortunately too familiar:

1. *Intrusive* feelings/thoughts
2. *Avoidance* of memory stimulations
3. *Negative* mood/thoughts
4. *Arousal*/reactivity elevation

The UCLA PTSD reactions index is 12 questions. A score over 21 leads to further evaluation and treatment (Pynoos et al., 2014).

And treatment. Two challenging words. We will discover in our children new approaches to treatment when faced with not only October 7, not only April 13 (the Iranian barrage) but also the ongoing threats from all sides. We can begin treatment with Pynoos and colleagues' well-validated approach which has seven components. While it is labeled, "cognitive behavioral therapy," most of these will be familiar to child therapists, particularly the focus on feelings. The steps are age dependent.

1. Psychoeducation about trauma and its effects;
2. Parenting skills: to manage their stress; improve parenting techniques;
3. Relaxation: teach child techniques to manage anxiety and stress;
4. Affective expression and regulation: *identify* and cope with *emotions*;
5. Cognitive coping: recognize/modify unhelpful trauma beliefs;
6. Trauma narrative: guide child narrative that recounts the trauma;

7. In-vivo mastery of trauma reminders: gradually expose the child to trauma reminders to reduce sensitivity (such as returning to the home); and
8. Child–parent sessions: facilitate effective communication.

I suggest supplementing the previous with child-created books illustrated and written by the children. With active supervision (therapist as "editor"), we can begin with two books: the book about today and the past; and the book about the future. We used this approach successfully in our Ethiopian children's study and piloted it in December with children near the October 7 catastrophe. A counselor would sit individually with each child giving prompts. We start with more neutral, house/tree/person. This would guide us to the more free-wheeling next portion. Draw a picture of October 7. Draw a picture of you on October 7. Tell me stories about each. Draw pictures about today and tell stories, and the second book is on stories about what you think the future will be like; what you hope the future will be for you. Depending on the child's responses, we would proceed following the child. Each book should be bound and given to the child as gift. The collection of books can be bound and with the child's permission, published so that other children can learn from them. But the aim of the book is to give the child a voice that she or he can listen to and that others (parents, teachers, peers) will also hear.

I end with this. Much simpler sounding. More concrete than our voyages with Odysseus Aeneus and Danté. Less harsh than the Hell of October 7. Yet more hopeful and, we believe, helpful to the children and the rest of us who wish to help children and parents emerge from Hell with greater wisdom on living a good life. If we use a *lev shomeah*, a heart that listens, and we act with an informed heart (Bettelheim, 1960), we can emerge from Hell on Earth to a better life for our children. Erikson described being a parent or grandparent as being like cogs on a wheel, a wheel that meshes the other wheels of children and grandchildren. Our task is to mesh so that both of us—parents/grandparents can move our children and they can move us toward a good life.

######

Notes

1 Perhaps Levi was twisting Pontius Pilates' pithier comment on Christ on the cross, "Ecco homo!" "Here is a man!"
2 Kings Book I, 3;9. God interpreted Shlomo's request as meaning, "To discern what is right" (Kings 3:11). This is a necessary component for a judge, as he showed in the tale of the two contending mothers. I thank my colleague, Ofra Eshel, for turning me to this phrase, a good one for a psychoanalyst (Szajnberg, N. 2019). *Book Review: The Emergence of Analytic Oneness: Into the Heart of Psychoanalysis*, Ed. Ofra Eshel. Routledge.
3 There were some 8,000 casualties in Beersheba's Soroka Hospital on October 7.
4 Despite the active filming by Hamas itself, the filming of headless babies or limbs and women's breasts amputated, women reaped to death, some still deny this was done by Hamas or that Palestinians either participated or celebrated these hours.

5 Three shoulder to shoulder, one at the feet. They rotated. The brothers' Yiddish joke was "Sleep quickly, we need the pillow."

6 Marshall, S. L. A. 1947. *Men Against Fire*. NY: Morrow, pp. 42–43.
   Stouffer, A. et al. 1949. *The American Soldier Combat and Its Aftermath* (Col. 2). Princeton University Press.

7 Wong, L., Kolditz, T., Millen, R., & Potter, T. 2003, July. Whey They Fight: Combat Motivation in the Iraqi War. *Global security.org*.

8 Burlingham, D., & Freud, Anna. 1949. *War Children*. London: Imago Publishing.

9 The Yiddish word for unkosher meat is *tref*, which is from the Hebrew *taref*, to tear an animal from limb to limb while still alive.

10 We note: tens of thousands protested in the streets against the government which was elected by some millions of Israelis. The minority (mostly Ashkenazi, secular Jews) seemed to have difficulty with accepting the majority rule (mostly Sephardi, more religious Jews). If I am correct, this is an old divide in Israeli society.

11 The photo on the cover of my book, *Reluctant Warriors*, pictures one such exhausted, drained soldier.

12 One terrorist "ingredient" is to hold a society hostage to fear. This must be countered actively.

13 I have shortened and edited Bennett's response.

14 Author's additions in parentheses.

15 Bettelheim, after spending a sabbatical in Japan, returned to note that Americans *talk* about feelings; Japanese act upon them.

16 These dogs are used to inspect houses or even tunnels.

17 Often on return, I would pick up soldier hitchhikers at the bus stop. (This was later prohibited by the Army after kidnappings of soldiers.) On one such stop, five strapping guys piled in. After dumping their duffels in the Prius's trunk, they squished in, their M16's nestled upright between their legs. I was likely the best-armed Prius in the Middle East.

18 Harold Kudler, MD., again I thank for this clarification.

References

Alighieri, D. 2003. *The Inferno*, Tr. John Ciardi. Penguin.

Bettelheim, B. 1960. *The Informed Heart*. Glencoe.

Bettelheim, B. 1979. *Surviving*. Knopf.

Freud, A. 1976. *Infants without Families Reports on the Hampstead Nurseries*. IUP.

Freud, A. and Burlingam, D. 1949. Anna Freud; *Collected Works*. Hogarth Press.

Gampel, Y. 1998. Reflections on Countertransference in Psychoanalytic Work with Child Survivors of the Shoah. *Journal of the American Academy of Psychoanalysis* 26: 343–368.

Grinker, R. 1945. *Men Under Stress*. McGraw Hill.

Horn, D. 2022. *People Love Dead Jews*. Norton.

Janowitz, M. 1960. *The Professional Soldier: A Social and Political Portrait*. Free Press.

Kafka, F. 2000. *The Penal Colony*. Schocken.

Laor, N. 2005. Personal Communication.

Lengyel, O. 1947. *Five Chimneys. The Story of Auschwitz*. Ziff-Davis.

Levi, P. 2015. *This is a Man*. Norton.

Minco, Margo. 1957. *Bitter Herbs*. Querido.

Pynoos, R. et al. 2014. Modeling Constellations of Trauma Exposure in the National Child Traumatic Stress Network Core Data Set. *Psychological Trauma: Theory, Research, Practice, and Policy* 6, No. S1: S9–S17.

Solomon, Z. 2008. In Waltz with Bashir, Dir. by Ari Folman. Sony.

Spencer, J. 2022. *Understanding Urban Warfare*. Howgate Publishing.
Stouffer, A. et al. 1949. *The American Soldier Combat and Its Aftermath* (Col. 2). Princeton University Press.
Szajnberg, N. M. 2006. *Reluctant Warriors: Israelis Between Rome and Jerusalem*. Amazon.
Szajnberg, N. M. 2013. *Sheba and Solomon's Return: Ethiopian Children in Israel*. Amazon.
von Clausewitz, C. 1832/1984. *On War*. Princeton University Press.
Wong, L. et al. 2003. *Why They Fight: Combat Motivation in the Iraq War*. Strategic Studies Institute, US Army War College.

3 The Children of Our Dreams

Antidotes to Despair

Refreshing to visit the evacuated children of Kibbutz Erez who since October 7, live in nearby Kiryat Gat apartments, just now, some parents are moving back to the Kibbutz, which we later visited with the psychologist, S. We stopped in three classrooms: under two, two to four, and four to six years. The atmosphere was a calm "busyness" and the staff, a hovering presence. It was delightful when the older kids (in the outside playground) took us on "tour." One was mixing "concrete" to build a building. Two others poured in sand or water as the mixer used a flayed, beaten-up, oversized whisk to stir patiently. One girl stands by, narrating the process for my sake; the master mixer and his assistants offer clarifying interjections. Surrounding us is the most popular area of the playground, the house discards populated the area—old pans, inoperable microwaves, pots, oversized utensils—beyond which were beaten-up chairs. This could be a visual and physical metaphor for our task at hand; how to reuse and remake an active life from the battered remains of almost discards.

The *metaplot*, the nursery teachers, wear their pedagogy softly, as if conducting with a baton, no, a magic wand, as the children perform the cantatas of their lives. In fact, in one classroom, the under fours, a music/ movement teacher was singing and conducting with her hands as the children joined in. I confess that I too joined the fun. Not conducting, but rather dancing hand movements which the children imitated. Only one girl of the eight seemed hesitant as she looked at us (in the back) with some stranger anxiety. Yet after a few minutes, she—keeping her eyes on me— blossomed and danced toward me, just a bit, before she retreated to her teacher's side. It was a touching *pas-de-deux*, in which my "steps" were to stand still, moving hands only, singing only, and casting occasional glances toward her until our eyes met briefly; then she released herself to the music and dance.

In the five- to six-year-old classroom, the movement teacher set some paint buckets upside down in a row and invited children individually to traipse across, holding her hand, as the music played. Tiny tot Wallendas, they balanced with arms extended. Then, from her humongous bag, she rooted about "discovering" colored Nerf balls and rolling them softly to each child as she

DOI: 10.4324/9781003618690-4

called out the colors and they chorused in response. It was this ball that the once-recalcitrant girl rolled toward me, and I softly rolled back.

Il said, I liked pictures and stories by children. Then, a half-dozen kids scrum around a table getting paper and crayons. Their stories are compelling, revealing, and hopeful. These stories and pictures will become the child's individual book and provide a guide to self-healing. These would be books of their past, the momentary present (like Heraclitus' flowing stream), to future hopes. I used a similar technique with the Ethiopian 9- and 11-year-olds in Kiryat Malachi. I knew that visiting and spending time with these preschoolers would be an antidote to despair: their lively activity, their sense of feeling safe and being protected, bring hope and remind us of what our future is and can be. I'd suggest that all members of the Kibbutz spend perhaps a half-day weekly with the children. A form of "treatment" for the child; gratifying for the therapist; relief for the parents.

From these exiled children in Kiryat Gat, I visited their now-repopulating Kibbutz Erez. This is near the infamous Erez Crossing from which terrorist *nukhba* swarmed by truck and paraglider-suspended motorcycles, bristling with arms. At the end of my visit, I stood on the ridge overlooking the murder road from Gaza into Kibbutz *Nitivot Asarah*, which suffered many more dead than *Erez*. Today, in *Erez*, there is a small cohort of Australian Amish who have moved to this Kibbutz for some months to help paint, rebuild the Kibbutz. I saw the old children's house, with a bowed steel roof pierced by rockets, being built (not rebuilt, but built anew) because the rockets had shredded the old building's steel. The new children's house, in contrast to Kibbutz life open to the land, will be safer, but closed-in, windows small, and double-walled exteriors (like Masada). The kibbutzniks feel a claustrophobic loss of freedom for their children. But the need to protect the children is foremost. Later, one of the kibbutzniks detailed the covered walkways and buses for the children, emphasizing the moments of vulnerability on their trips to school. Just some 15 seconds from Red Alert to get the children to safety. Safety? If they are on the school bus, the children must leave it, hit the ground face down, mouth open, legs crossed, and arms overhead along the road's edge.

But back to the concrete mixers in Kiryat Gat. Following their account of their future building, I invite them to sit to draw pictures and tell stories. Often, when I meet individually with children, I ask them to draw a person, tree, house, and family doing something. Here, with the group of eight crowding around the table, I ask them to draw anything that "comes to them" (*ba lecha/ lach*). Then, I ask for a story from each. Not able to curb their enthusiasm, I often got several reciting together and scribbled what I could in Hebrew on their pictures. I wish the reader could see *how* spontaneous their drawings were and how rich their stories were. These children are internally poised (*mutzav*, in Hebrew) to tell their most personal stories through pictures and "pretend" stories; about fears, yes, but more so about their wishes.

I'll begin with "Elah"[1] but interrupt with others' pictures and stories. I do so, because, Elah kept drawing,[2] pausing, considering her picture, continuing,

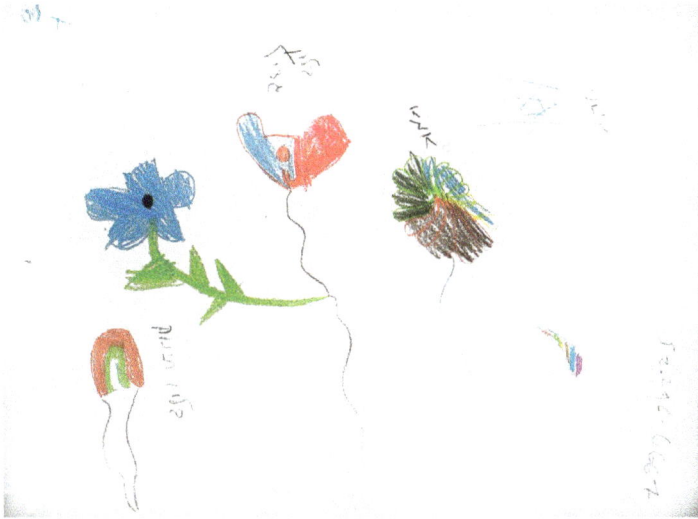

Figure 3.1 "Elah's" Balloon Family.

then editing, and revising at the end. A film of her work would be more revealing than the final static picture (Figure 3.1).

In lieu of the film, I will describe her process. Five-year-old Elah begins by carefully articulating three sets of five overlapping petals of a flower; each petal looks like a curved tadpole, its tail rooting it to the center and to each other. Each petal carefully spoons into another. Each set of five is a different color. This flower is at the center of the paper. She works meticulously, slowly, occasionally pausing to reflect on what she's done. Others dashed off their pieces, a couple of boys doing treasure maps with gold at the end and even "instructions" on how to get through the mazes. Then, Elah bows her head to continue. At times, her tongue tip peeks through her lips as she concentrates. She draws a wiggly line from the flower to the bottom of the paper, its stem. Then she adds four more figures, balloons, she says. One is "tethered" with its stem to the ground; another is tethered with a thick green stem to the second balloon; the fourth balloon, an Israeli flag balloon, has a string that doesn't reach to the ground, but is held down by a colorful simple figure, like a comma, or a tadpole inverted. There is inherent tension potential energy in a tethered balloon—straining for the sky, while tied to the ground; in a word, "*nitzav*" poised for action.[3] Finally, on the far left is a "baby balloon" that has no string by whose head has a green-blue core capped with a red top. The balloons are colored in. The big balloon is half blue and half red, with a visible red eye and half smile in the blue and the other half smile/eye colored over by the red. At the end, she rather furiously scribbles colors on the first meticulously drawn petals, using a dun brown to scribble over the one-third that were bright orange petals. The other two-thirds are also colored, but by the same colors of the petals, less obscured. Asked for a story, she mentions that she has a new baby brother, a few weeks old (conceived around the time of October 7). Elah names the figures. From our right, the Israeli flag anchored by the multicolored upside-down comma is a balloon. Next, the central multi-petaled figure is mommy. Then is big balloon, with half face blue, half red, and the next figure a blue flower tethered to big balloon's stem. Finally on the left and near the bottom is baby balloon, of sperm-like or tadpole shape. When Elah scribbled over the mother's one-third of her face, I felt the urge to halt her, not to spoil the delicate petals (of course, I did not do this, permitting her will). She seemed depleted after all this effort. We can speculate here about Elah's story-free associations. She tells us that the central figure is a mother flower balloon. Its face is made of three sets of five petals: we know that Elah is five years old and that her brother was born recently. (The midwives at Soroka Hospital informed me that there was a burst of child-births in the months following October 7; assertions of life.)

We also can speculate that the original mother flower face consists of three sets of petals, as there were originally three in her family: mother father and herself. The brownish scribble overlaying the mother's lower face leads us to wonder if her newborn brother has brought some darkness and some sadness to her mother. This sadness, if we read her correctly, *may also be* the attack on October 7 and the aftermath of dislocation. Children's logic is simple and a concatenation of proximal events—October 7; pregnancy; move to a new home—may be confounded in the child. In any case, the trajectory of her story is one of colorful beginning shifting to a shadowing of her joy.

Ariel draws a Mondrian-like geometric treasure map.

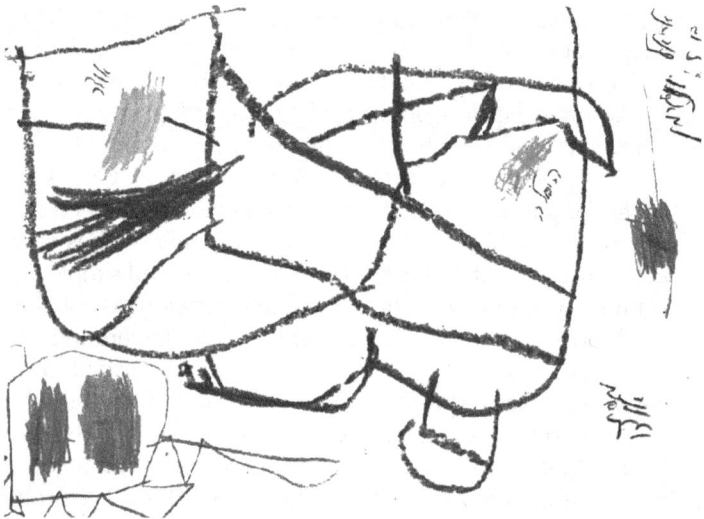

Figure 3.2 Ariel's Mondrian-Like Treasure Map With Instructions.

He clearly marks the treasure in the upper left and gives scribbled instructions on how to get through the maze as well as a starting point; all three of these markers are orange. While the maze is complex, his instructions at the start and the bright and shiny treasure offer hope in the end.

Ofek also makes a maze with treasure embedded. He explains that one must skip through this maze (a joyful way to move through life). The starting point is a scribble of circles with a looped line leading into the mostly rectangular maze, obscured with brown circle blobs and ending with a series of interconnected pinkish drips before the treasure outside the maze.

Baruch's portrait is simple: a figure with a large round head–body, two eyes, and two legs. There is no nose or mouth or arms, suggesting a more infantile figure who cannot speak or manipulate the world about him.

Reuven is the youngest in the group, 4.5. He draws a simple orange right-angle triangle at the bottom left and a rectangle atop. It is a bridge connecting to a balloon.

Finally, we have Micah, a little girl who has an eye for design. She uses bold colors:

> charcoal, purple, blue, green—to make a blouse made in the style of a balloon. Perhaps the charcoal at the heart of the design suggests some darkness in her own center, but the colorful sleeves and bottom offset these.

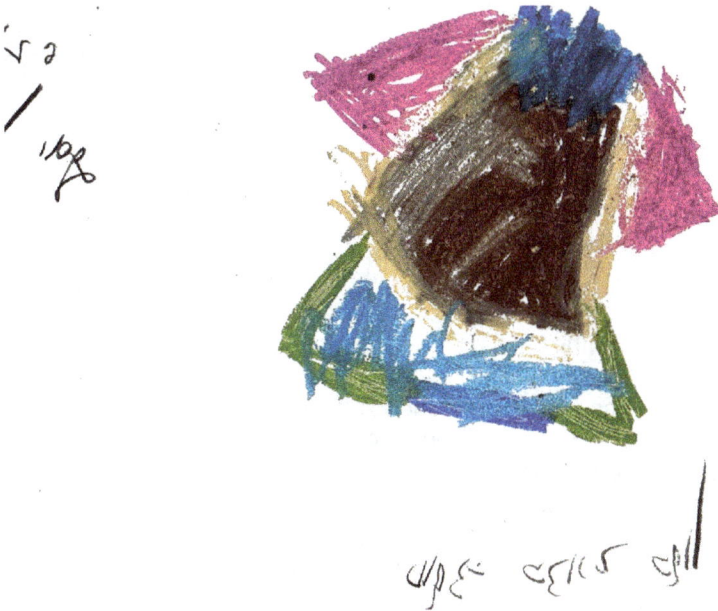

Figure 3.3 Balloon Blouse.

Before we turn to the slightly older Ethiopian children, what can we learn from these portraits/stories? For they are "portraits/stories"' of their inner lives. We have only their brief stories and pictures, no clinical background or a formal interview. But, like Donald Winnicott (1974), we can take these brief initial encounters and the story/free associations as unfettered glimpses into their lives. Overall, these children are remarkably free about creating, both drawing and telling. It takes little encouragement, only a request, for them to set about creating. The details of their creations suggest their very personal "take" on life. Treasure will be found if one follows their complex mazes (instructions included); colors predominate, even if some colors are darkened by shadows; and Elah's painstakingly detailed story has both hope—the floating balloons, the family of balloons—and some hint of shadows—mother's partly obscured colored petals and the sperm-like baby balloon lurking at the periphery. We cannot for certain say that October 7 overshadows these children; we might speculate that the four- and five-year-olds pick up the shadows of their parents or *metapellets'* preoccupation with October 7 and their temporary dislocation from home. What we do return to is our overall sense of the hopeful, calm, and busyness of this preschool. It would be a fine antidote to despair and a tincture of future for all adults to spend time in this preschool. Yes, a prescription, at least one "dose" per week.

And Now We Are Nine: Ethiopian/Israeli Children

A preface. Between 2007 and 2010, I worked with and learned from Ethiopian six-year-olds in Elie Wiesel's Beit Tzipporah after school in Kiryat Malachi. I wrote a book, *Sheba and Solomon's Return* (Szajnberg, 2013), about their lives, their pictures and stories, and their parents, all of whom immigrated from Ethiopia. My last research assistant, Zehava (Yeshi in Ethiopian, which means "Goldie") is the mother of four (quadruplets) and a fifth older son. We have remained in touch and she now teaches at Beit Tzipporah. So, returning to "my kids" was something I anticipated with wonder and excitement and some trepidation: they are in rocket distance of Gaza; they were not attacked, but on my visit in December, the principal, Moshe Shateh, said that when the red alert sirens sounded, the children began crying: they feared not for themselves but for their older brothers and fathers and uncles and aunts who were in the army. In fact, Anna Freud and colleagues (Freud and Dann, 1951) found that during the V-bombing of London, those children whose mothers showed greater calm did better than those whose mothers showed overt fear. Zehava's five children are now serving: four in Gaza, one in (slightly less dangerous, slightly) Hebron: the latter daughter is a (well-armed) cook. I used to drive my Toyota Prius from Jerusalem down to Kiryat Malachi, an hour-plus trip. On the way back, I'd stop at the bus stand to pick up soldiers heading home either to Jerusalem or en route. On one such memorable return, four soldiers piled into my silver Prius, first hiking their rucksacks into the trunk, then sitting with their rifles erect between their knees. They marveled at the then-new touchscreen and controls for music. I joked that I was likely the best-armed Prius in the Middle East. (Later, because of soldier kidnappings, it was prohibited to give soldiers rides. I missed this.)

But That Was Then, What About Now?

In the cab down, we hunted for the unnumbered address, and I had slight concern I wouldn't recognize the set-back building. But there it was. It looked a bit worn from age and the Mediterranean sun. I knew that the funds Wiesel had set aside from his writing for the School were evaporated (Ponzi-stolen) by Bernie Madoff.[4] The security guard was once a Moroccan with a gun holstered as he sat and read *Tehillim* (psalms) on the five steps leading up to the door. I saw no guard today. The kids would arrive at 130 or so and I was early enough to enter the unusually quiet, central atrium with Greek-style semi-circular steps facing a stage. Here, the whole school would gather for plays or songs or just for fun. The backyard was for breaks; the yellowed grass was beaten down by the sun and children's soccer games. But Zehava descended with her usual smile and warm embrace and prepared a quiet classroom for me next to hers to meet with the children. Moshe Shateh had a powerful glass of coffee for me—*botz* (mud) it is called in Israel, often served with the spice of *hel*, cardamom. (He'd just returned from army service in Gaza.) He was looking for a therapist last December, when I visited and I offered to find someone. But today, he told me that he had found a psychologist to meet with the kids and parents; in fact she was the former principal, an Ethiopian. Upstairs I knew I had four hours to meet with the children. Meeting with them individually and with more time than in Kiryat Gat, I asked each to draw anything they wanted, then a picture of a person, then the person of the opposite gender, a tree, a house, and a family doing something (also known as the HTP). This was familiar from my last work with the kids and proved useful today. I had no information about each child except what they revealed to me.

I could have done Winnicott's Squiggle Game but chose this more structured event of the House-Tree-Person (HTP Buck, 1977).

A: The house weakened by magic, abandoned, then regained.

A. is a nine-year-old girl who began with a stick figure man with round face, smile, and dot eyes. His clothes are two rectangles with short sleeves. Her story?

"One man walked and saw his friend. Both were good friends and so they went to enjoy an evening together and they laughed, and it was fun for them. And this was enjoyment for them. The end."

Then she drew a girl with long, long hair. When I remark on this, she draws it longer, past her waist, and flipped over to her left. She too has a stick figure, round face, and smile, but the eyes are now circles and a tiny nose appears. She wears pants and blouse, both rectangles. If we look between her legs, she has a long extension that runs past her feet, a penis, one might speculate, continuous with her spine.

A girl walked to the play garden and saw her classroom (female) friend. And then she said, "Don't laugh at me." And she said, "Good." They both walked and laughed together and that's the end.

Her house has a door, and two windows, one of which is filled in with a square and decoration. Both windows have scribbles above them, like eyebrows. She calls them sunshades (like those outside of windows to block the fierce sun). Under the roof are stairs that go up. The windows are like wide-set eyes and the obscured; shadowed left eye reminds us of Picasso's early portrait of himself, one eye blackened. Her story was elaborate and telling.

It's a pretty house that was sold and the house was sad. A new person came, but the house was weakened by magic. Good. And then she sold the house and the house was sad. And then the house was returned to someone who was the first owner. The end.

Her tree has a somewhat squat trunk, substantial crown and four thick roots, two large and two smaller. "This tree, *she* is tall and *he* (sic) will have a good life. And then they killed him and he died. But, there remained roots and then the tree grew anew and he had a new life."

Her family are four stick figures, all with three "legs" the middle one longest, except the brother, who has only two legs (and a slight branch off one). The mother is the biggest with a cascade of long hair over her left side; father is smaller, as is sister (also with a cascade of locks to her feet and brother). All smile. This family was wealthy. And then the family went on a field trip to America. And they went to life there. And they were happier. The end. She wants to draw one more picture and does a stick figure of a girl with the familiar third overly long leg, herself, and two small girlfriends. After she draws her cascade of long, smooth hair, she admits that she wants this for herself. (Her hair is in a short bun and very curly.) She draws a square shirt and skirt. Her story is brief, a wish. The shirt is "An *Eli Cohen* shirt. My mother or father will buy it for me."

We can listen and look at her drawings both individually and as a series of snapshots of a narrative. Both her man and girl persons find fun with a friend; although the girl's friend seems catty at first, she changes to playful. It is more typical for boys and girls to draw a person of their own gender at first. That this girl draws a man first and in later pictures, portrays girls, mom (and dad, but not brother) with a third middle leg (a penis, we might speculate), suggests that this girl finds "strength" in some male identification. The pretty house is abandoned by its beloved owner because magic weakens the house. After an interval with a new owner, the original one returns.

The tree had a good life, and is cut down but, because of its strong roots, regrows. The family starts wealthy but finds a new land where it is happier. A narrative thread is one being cut down or sold or weakened by magic, but a hopeful ending, particularly if one has strong roots. Let's leave this modest interpretation for now and turn to our next child.

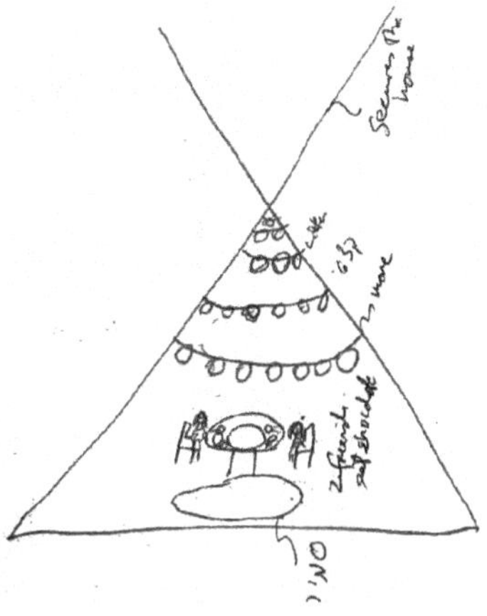

Figure 3.4 Or's Teepee House With Two Girls Having Chocolate.

Or: The tree with teethy leaves.

"Or" starts off with a spontaneous house that is an X (or exaggerated teepee shaped).

Two girls sit in the lower triangle opposite each other with a round table between that has two legs and food. A cover (*smicha*) is under the table. Above the girls are strung five tiers of lights, like a necklace (which she calls, *"keshet" or rainbow*).

"Two friends eating chocolate. The top part of the X secures the house." She draws a girl first with long hair on both sides and darkened eyes, a pupil peeking in the lower quadrant. She has stick arms and legs but a full body and skirt. "She's sweet." Loves to take trips to the park to play with the boy "(next to her in the picture). She's 12." There is no story about the boy, except he's five. One eye appears deformed.

Her tree is unique.

It has a strong trunk that she later colors in to make bark, which covers the few sinuous, gentle lines beneath. Its branches are six very thin, sinuous lines that sprout what looks like canine teeth but are supposed to be leaves. On one branch are two or maybe four flowers, darkened ovals. The house begins with a left side that curves into a floor, but she says is an error. She draws a straighter line for the floor. She doesn't know what's inside. By her "family" picture, some dour mood has overtaken her. Or yet her family story tries to deny this apparent dourness. She draws a ten-year-old birthday girl with a crown; a mother holding her hand, then a tall six-layer cake in the middle with one candle, and then a six-year-old brother and next to him, father. "It's her birthday. She's happy." When I note that the cake has six layers and the brother is six, and I ask if something special happened when she was six, she responds "Nothing happened." And shuts down. When I first saw the cake, I thought it had four layers (the thick ones in the picture). But she corrected me that the two long rectangles on top of the four were not candles, but two

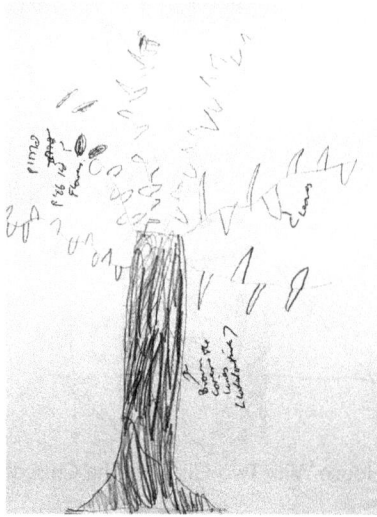

Figure 3.5 Or's Teethy Tree.

more layers. I thought to myself that she was four when her brother was born, but nearing the end of our meeting didn't pursue this.

Eidan: Falling Tree, Weeping Boy

Eidan's person is first a girl with a triangle dress, smile, and stick limbs.

> Once some children from class made on her a *cherem* (an excommunication), because she that she thought of her self as a fun queen. The children made an excommunication because of this thing. Only after some in the class were for me and helped, then I didn't care if the other children made a *cherem* on me.

A boy stick figure with a broad smile. "One day I walked to play. We played tag. I was the tagger and there were several others to play with and then I succeeded to tag." The house is a simple square with a triangular roof, two windows, and an arch-top door with a handle in the middle. "Once, the parents started to build a home. They looked for a long time. It was good, got solid. They went to a new house. They arranged that everything went well in the end. A fun life." He adds, "I have two brothers 13, 6 and three sisters 5, 3 and 1 and Mommy is 33; daddy is 40."

Eidan's tree (not shown here) is a stout rectangular trunk and squiggly crown.

> Not so good (he refers to his drawing). Once one a day, my parents buy for me a tree to grow. I planted and I had the responsibility to water it.

One day, it falls, and I cried like it was my life. My parents said no worry, well get another one. I said it's not the same as the old and I cried. Bought a new one. I didn't want to plant it because it would fall down like the old. In the end, he planted it and it was better than the old.

I ask about anyone falling down in his life.

On Wednesday, my great grandmother fell and died. She was sick (My grandmother always played with my shoes.) The family is a father, brother, sister and mother all stick figures with square hands with little squares in the palms. They are playing cards. Search for a card and discover what the other cards are. Whoever gets the most wins. Father won. Got a prize. A phone.

He drew a picture of the future, a frowning fellow facing two different schools.

A guy who's sad because he must leave his school, Etzion, and go to Netzach. But he will miss his friends. In reality, his mother asked him to change schools and he said no and she listened. The tree story is compelling: what his parents once gave him, he tended, yet it still fell.

While his parents want to "repair" or "compensate," *Eiden* is honest: it will (he will) never be the same. But a reality principle sets in as he plants and it is good. His house story shares a similar theme: his parents searched for a long time and found a good house. And his "future" story and more importantly his associations also carry the significant theme that his mother listened to him about not changing schools: that friends were important too. All in all, Eiden sees a future of realistic hope: things may fall down (and unlike his great grandmother, but like his tree) and can regrow. He trusts his parents.

Chazit: Born crippled, but "It doesn't bother him."

Chazit's boy person has a full torso, stick arms with hands and fingers a round face with a broad smile, widened eyes and uplifted eyebrows and . . . dotted legs.

"A man who likes to travel around the world. He always takes with him
someone important to him. So that he will be busy with him."
(His legs?)
"He was born like this, but it doesn't bother him."
(She shows no deformity and denies having one.)

She draws a stick girl with full A-line skirt and blouse. She too has a smile, widened eyes, raised eyebrows, and hands bristling with fingers.

A girl who loves to play one game. She really wanted everyone to play with her. But not everyone loves this game that she loves so much. And once

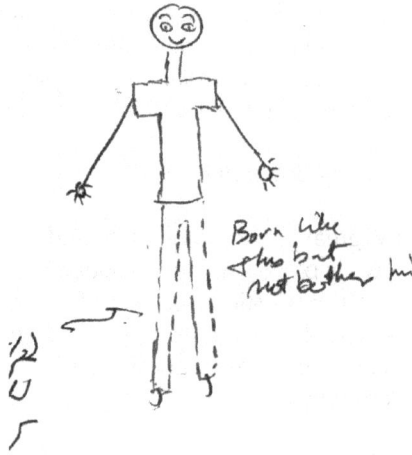

Figure 3.6 Chazit's Dotted-Legged Crippled Man.

one of the children (a boy) came and said to her, "Stop playing this game." She felt quite sad because they shouted at her. But she didn't remain sad. She prepared a game that was quite interesting and then she returned to her classroom what she found. And everyone in the end played together.

Chazit draws a simple house with widespread windows; the door has a defect at its lower corner.

One day two children went to school and suddenly they saw a house. This house didn't have anything, not a thing. The two children entered the house. They saw that the house was filthy with dust and suddenly they heard a loud sound they saw a old man and they ran out and we're frightened and really ran from this house and never came back again.

Her tree has a hefty lumpy crown atop a feathery light trunk with a flat base, no roots visible.

One day there was a boy and he loved trees. But he really loved the most of all the trees, this tree. He loved to be next to the tree and to draw. One day the boy returned from school. He saw that people were cutting down the tree. And the boy said "No! Don't cut down this tree!" One man said, "We must cut down the tree. And plant something new." And the boy argued with them and didn't permit them to cut down the tree. The people said, "We will wait and return. And after this, we will cut down the tree." And the boy said "No, you *won't* cut it down, the tree on the street. You won't cut down the tree and in the end, the tree remained and they didn't cut it down."

Her family drawing is a mother, a boy, and an unnamed father. All the characters have some incomplete defect at the top of the head, covered by hair. Father's left leg is "defective"; drawn, erased, redrawn. "They play cards and watch a movie. But I can't draw that part."

Her future drawing is of her own Bat Mitzvah: Mother, Chazit, father all almost equal in size. "My future is that I will have a bat mitzvah in two years."

Tiglit: From Face to faceless— "I have no more strength."

Tiglit looks large for her nine years, tall and hefty. She begins with a delicately sketched girl's face and head. "This is my Bestie (best friend). She has already left and I yearn for her."

She makes finely drawn closed eyes and elegant eyelashes, a button nose, and small pursed lips. Next, she draws her aunt.

"She died last year. They did surgery because there was something in her throat and the illness was terrible."

(Dr. S "I see she has an empty face.")

"I feel *beseder* (fine, OK)."

(DR. S: you sound sad, though.) (She nods in assent.)

For the boy/male, she draws as she recites, that she left Ethiopia at two years old with her mother but left a brother behind. She draws another empty face with curly hair.

"My eldest brother (*ben habachor*, literally, "the chosen son"). I've been searching for him, because he was left in Ethiopia and I and my mother left the family and I yearn for him." She draws another empty-faced male. "My second brother. I also miss him.":

(DR. S: These sound like sad stories.) Tiglit reacts with withdrawal and an irritated look. She begins to shut down.

The house is lightly sketched, with a round-topped door and handle on the left. The windows are lightly sketched; the rooftop is cut off at the edge of the page.

"Happy. I and father and mother and little brother, who's six. My father came to Israel first."

Her Tree is a think stem-like trunk with an almost facial sketch and looping branches. "It's a nice, quiet place and happy to be there."

Her family is rapidly sketched, simple stick figures with empty circle faces and all have a third limb between the legs. A "sun" rises above with four cilia-like radiations and two wavy lines in the sky. The family floats above a wavy ground, and there is a light single dot between the legs. She dashes off quickly,

"Dad, mother, me and little brother." She says, "I have no strength to draw the faces." She seems short and irritated as we finish. My comment on the sad stories appeared to have distanced her.

And Now We Are Eleven

For some children, my time was restricted, so I could not do the more extensive house/tree/person/family. Instead, I asked them to draw, *"Mah sheh ba
lecha/lach."* "Whatever comes to you."

Silat drew a plumpish carrot with a crown, it is orange but is shaped more
like a radish.

> She's the king or queen who rules over all the carrots. It's ok that it's
> eaten, because can grow more. Once there was a rabbit that loved
> to eat carrots and who waits for the carrots to grow. It's not patient.
> He wants for a long time for the carrot to grow. He starts to be angry.
> Until once until he saw the tip of the carrot and he starts to be happy
> and the waits more until he sees the whole carrot. More rabbits came
> and they were hungry and the rabbit and the rabbits eat the car-
> rot and then more are waiting and he understands the meaning of
> waiting.

Chen is shy. She sits with her fingertips on her mouth, tight-lipped. She
draws a large red heart and above it, a small house with a single window
and a triangular roof set askew. The door is drawn as an afterthought. She
gives no story, except to say that the house is full of love. She adds that she
likes to play soccer, father doesn't work and mother does, and she has two
sisters.

Moriya makes a house with two askew windows in the roof—one for her,
the other for two brothers—and beneath the roof, a lower-quartered window
in the upper corner of the wall. No door is visible. It stands on a firm grassy
lawn and next to it is a flower, half the height of the house, with a red-lobed
flower. Floating above the flower and the house is a red heart. Beneath the
window is a *mirpesset*, a patio, that leads into the garden of *sha'ashuim* (of
children's toys).

> I really like my house. I live five minutes away from here. It doesn't look
> like this (She lives in a flat, like every child in Beit Tzipporah.) I have
> three rooms, also a computer room and two brothers and a sister. I'm
> the oldest with responsibilities to keep: the house, watch my brothers.
> I love my house and my family.

Itamar draws a solid blue Israeli flag with a star of David embedded. (I'm
told that many children are drawing the star of David since October 7.) "Israel
will be 76 in a bit. The is the symbol of my country. I feel happy. It is a strong
country. All the people like the country of Israel, love it. All the land. We will
win the war."

He adds that he's the oldest and has two sisters. His uncle has five sisters.
He identifies with this uncle.

"I help them (his sisters) with anything they need, like helping on tests."

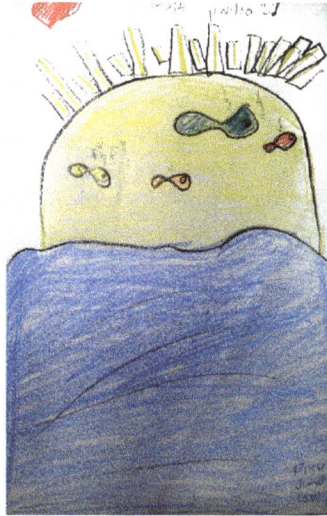

Figure 3.7 Lini's Fish Family Seeking Father.

Lini works avidly on a colorful picture the bottom half is a blue sea; the top, the sun as if emerging from the sea, is brightly yellow.

In front of the sun are four fish. A large blue one with a slight protrusion from the head and a smudged black eye is the mother, the leader. In front of the leader is a small red son; below the mother is another peach boy, and lagging behind is a small yellow fish with black outlines so it stands out from the sun. The latter is sick or lazy and is hidden in the sea. The jumping fish. The father is in the water (invisible). They are going to meet the father in the water at home. They jump to meet him. They are in the heart of God. They are going to find the father. When the sun sets, it is most beautiful. My father is at home. He finished a course and got a diploma.

(More about the sun?)

"The rays are strong."

In his external reality, he has four siblings. His wish at the end is for all the hostages to be healthy and return. Is his portrayal of a sea-hidden father also his wish for those captive fathers in Gaza? The mother and baby fish hope to be reunited with him when they return home. We would need to listen to him more to confirm this.

Tahal draws a forest of four trees with different colored fruit. A blue sky, ribbons just overhead, and a glimmering yellow sun is in the right corner. The trees stand firmly on grassy hillocks.

There's a forest with trees with red apples and fruits and vegetables. More people will come and grow more trees. All can take whatever they want. Their friends and family. You can make it a garden and make it whatever you want, like a swing.

Natanel draws two figures: one more typically head, torso, arms, and a bulging underwear for his oversized penis; the other is made of angular squares, a triangle, and one leg.

> This is one person. He met a girl with a square head. He bumped into her accidentally. She said, "What do you want?" He: "Sorry. It was an accident." She, "I forgive you" But, she hit him with her big head *first*.
>
> (Dr. S: She has one leg?)

"Oh, the other leg is broken from when she fell on the street. (Her square head) makes her look strange to him."

Hodiya is a delicate-looking girl who draws what looks like a black and green butterfly but in fact is a complex figure made up of significant others and herself. She then draws an Israeli flag in the upper corner. This is a friend and Hodiya. The center (black heart) is *Odiya*. (The black heart is drawn over a green central body.) The overall is Hodiya. Priel is one wing. They play dodgeball with a sponge ball (so it doesn't hurt). I usually win (she smiles).

"I have three sisters and a brother, 12, 16, 18 and the eleven-month-old who looks and acts like me."

Ilai draws a figure with round head/body and legs emerging from it, with arms. (This is more like the head/body drawn by a 3–4 year old.) He's smiling and has curly brown hair atop a blue figure. Four faint clouds and sun are above.

A man with eyes and nose and smile and feet and shoes, hands and hair. He's happy. He thinks thoughts: "I want to go outside tomorrow to play with friends."

(And?)

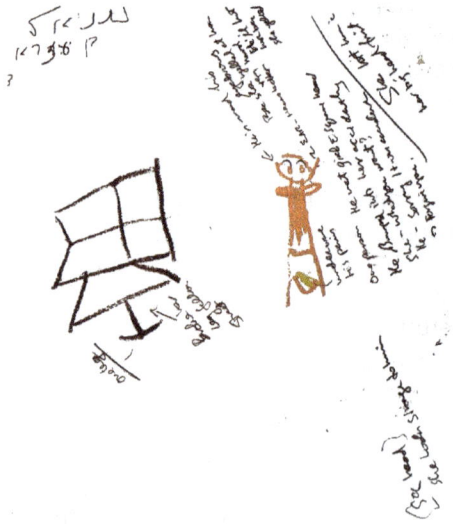

Figure 3.8 Natanel's Boy and Square-Headed One-Legged Mean Lady.

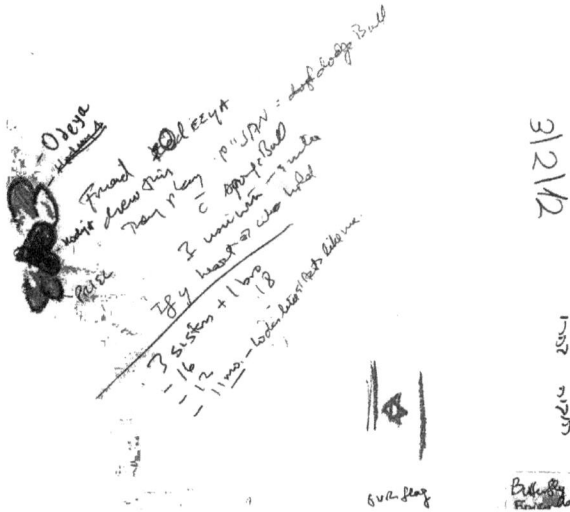

Figure 3.9 Two-Colored Butterfly on Left; Orange Wings and Black Body. Israel Flag on Right.

"It's too hot outside. Just go tomorrow. Play with my friend, Osher."

(Why is he smiling?) He tells jokes. (Clouds?) "Make the day The sun is in the morning and the clouds come in the evening. The sun will go down. The clouds go to cry rain. His hair will get wet. He's excited about the rain. He loves it."

We note how her figure appears like a butterfly, but it is composed of the central (black) Hodiya, and her wings are her two friends, suggesting that she feels both whole and able to fly with her friends as wings.

Omer draws a house with two quartered windows and a very wavy tiled roof (suggesting thinking going on). Previous is an unusual rainbow with five colors, anchored on each end with clouds.

"He came from a house from a place and half to one year moved to a house on the land. Much nicer. Thank God. Problems in the building on the second floor and its hard to lift bags."

(Rainbow?)

The sun plus the rain make it very pretty. The rainbow is interesting. The roof has like waves and in the backyard, you can play soccer. If there's no rainbow, then the clouds are separate and lonely. The rainbow makes them feel better. (Who's the rainbow?) "I'm the connection between *ima* and *aba* (mother and father)."

He adds that he has three sisters and five brothers (note the five colors of the rainbow, perhaps). Mother and father work. It's noisy at home.

I'm the youngest, and it's fun. I worry that when I return from the playground, I worry that in the house will have fights with siblings. I hit them back; then I get punished by not being permitted to go outside.

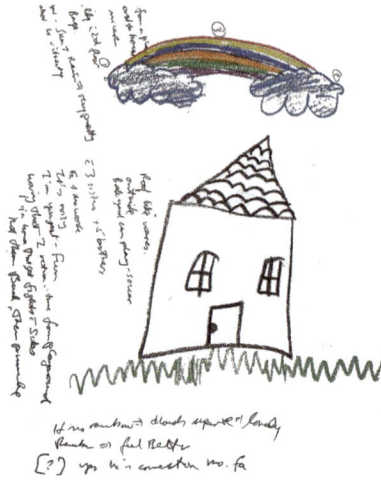

Figure 3.10 Colored Rainbow With Blue Clouds Over House With Shingled Roof.

Let's listen and learn from these children. They will lead us.

But first, *my* intrusive thought, one that I've never had in all my decades working with, listening to, children. As I was sitting with Elah, to my right, looking into her glistening blue eyes, her bouncy, curly blond hair, I thought, "She too, she would have been slaughtered by Hamas. As would these other children surrounding me." This felt like a smack in the back of my head. But this is precisely how the terrorist hopes to insinuate into our daily lives, to bore into our consciousness. Our task—even those like myself thousands of miles removed from October 7—is to defeat the terrorists' attempt to own us, hijack our inner lives. *After all, this is* **my** *intrusive thoughts; I can revise, diminish, transform my thoughts. This became a theme in my work with the Israelis: regaining autonomy, "self (internal) rule" in the Greek.*

I hope you will see and hear how these children are so ready, so prepared, to express their innermost, their most sincere thoughts. They will display themselves to us, if only we listen. If only we are not afraid of what they have to say. But what they have to say to us, overall, is a sense of hopefulness about their futures. These children expect us to protect them to let them live and fulfill their wishes: a new house; a tree will grow if cared for and *if* it falls (or is felled) will be regrown; that a child can be the rainbow that binds mother and father together; a house, once lived, then abandoned, will mourn until the original owner returns with love. *These displaced children will return to their Otef homes (or at least figuratively to their families before October 7) and the children will bring joy to their abodes.* And, intriguingly, there was little about *October 7* (overtly; unconscious fears will insinuate themselves). For the most part, many of these children can express more personal concerns about their home settings. And, as a psychoanalyst, when I hear personal concerns expressed, this is a moment of courage (from *coeur*, something from the heart): courage in which hope is embedded—if I express my concerns, someone will find a way to reassure me. Israeli parents (and government) should listen to these children. (The parents do; I ask to listen with a third ear.) They will lead us to better decisions, for them, and of course for ourselves as we care for them.

I present you pictures and stories from 5-, 9-, and 11-year-olds. Most are from children displaced from the Gaza envelope *yishuvim*; others are Ethiopian/Israeli children in Kiryat Malachi, a town not invaded (fortunately), but whose children hear the red alarm, whose fathers, brothers, and uncles (and aunts) are fighting, protecting them, in Gaza. For instance, look at Omer, the boy rainbow connecting mother and father. As a psychoanalyst, I speculate that he is the binding element that holds the (possibly arguing) mother and father together. And poetically, a rainbow is made of both rain and sun: tears and happiness, such as he may feel as the colorful arc keeping them together. Omer not only says he's happy as the youngest but also confesses that when there are fights at home, he gives back as much as he gets and he gets punished. All this is normal for a big family. The Chinese have a saying, "No family can hang a sign outside their home that says, 'No troubles here.'" Yes, troubles, but manageable.

Let's return to Elah's meticulous picture and story of the 15-petaled flower (mother) accompanied by balloons of father and brother and little baby (who has no tethering stem unlike the others). Elah is surrounded by (mostly boys), who dash off Minotaur mazes with treasures at the end and even instruct *us* how to navigate the maze (of their lives). We can say here that for many of these four-, five-, and six-year-olds, their lives may feel maze like, but they also feel that there is a pot of gold at the end. And they even have formulae for how to negotiate the maze; like Jason, they have their own Ariadne's.

But Elah tells a more complex tale, one that she spins out over time, then harshly, radically revises. At the epicenter of her family portrait is *Ima*, mother, the first to appear. Elah returns to *Ima* repeatedly to revise as she fills in balloons of Janus-faced father (alongside mother), a blue-flowered flower (girl) balloon rooted to the father's stem; a balloon Israel flag (anchored by stem and a sperm-like, multicolored organelle). She concentrates in the beginning on making each *Ima* petal spoon against another, in a trio of colors (as if to represent her original family before October 7 and before the pregnancy: mother father and herself). Notice that only the *Ima* stem is closest to being grounded; the others are afloat. After all the other characters are drawn, she returns to the "face" of the *Ima* flower, first obscuring two of the trio of petals with scribbles of the same hue, then finishes by rather fiercely obscuring the pink petals with brown scribbles. We can speculate here and would need to spend more time with Elah, deciphering the details. Two-thirds of mother's face remains colorful, even if the margins of the petals are obscured; the third part of her face is darkened. The timing gives us some clues. It is nine months since October 7; Elah's baby brother is recently born. Does the mother's dark face represent the darkening of October 7 and mirrored in mother's face? Does it represent (to Elah) the darkening of her life since baby brother's birth? Does she conflate the tragedies/displacement of October 7 with mother's pregnancy? Such conflation can take place in the simple logic of children's minds. Does the Elah balloon's tethering to the father balloon's stem suggest that Elah can anchor herself in safety when connected with her father? In any case, Elah gives us clues of what to pursue with her and how to untether her mind from such concerns.

What we wish to convey here is that our children will let us know their views of life, including October 7 and its aftermath, if we watch what they "say" in their play, their drawings, and their stories. But following their lead, we can begin to repair their trust in us and hence their world. We can, as Elah's cohort drew around her, help them navigate this maze of life to reach their pots of gold. We learn to listen with Solomon's *lev shomeah* to these children. But with their drawings they also teach us to see, but to see, in the Hebrew sense of *hitbonen, reflective* seeing/understanding.

With that, let us turn to the soldiers who protect these children. They too have tales to tell. Let us hear with and even develop a listening heart, *lev shomeah*, as King Solomon asked of God. ########

Notes

1 All names are fictionalized. But "Elah" is the valley where the shepherd David slew Goliath. Today, a tall TV tower stands. Once, a fox chewed through the cables beneath, slewing himself and casting TV sets around Israel into darkness.
2 One of my infancy teachers, Sally Provence, taught me this technique. Soft waiting, unobtrusive watching, patience, and waiting for the invitation to engage.
3 I thank Professor R. Alter, who taught me the three words for "stand" in Biblical Hebrew. "Kam" is to stand up; "Omed" is to stand; "Nitzav" is to stand poised for action, as was Joseph in his dreams (or the ladder in Jacob's dream).
4 Wiesel's "punishment" wish for Madoff was that Madoff should have cast on his cell wall the photos of all the children and people whom he'd robbed.

References

Buck, J. 1977. *HTP*. WPS Publishing.
Freud, A., & Dann, S. 1951. An Experiment in Group Upbringing. *Psychoanalytic Study of the Child* 6: 127–166.
Szajnberg, N. 2013. *Sheba and Solomon's Return: Ethiopian Children in Israel.* Amazon.

4   The IDF Soul Healers (Sde Teiman)

I was excited, anticipating meeting with the IDF (Israel Defense Forces) psychiatrists and psychologists and *kabanim* (mental health crisis interventionists) near the Gaza front at *Sde Teiman* base in the Negev. Lt. Col. Shai Neustadt, MD, is both on faculty at Soroka Hospital and in charge of the IDF Southern Command mental health services. He wears a *kippah srugah*, a "knitted" skullcap, which I recall is a signal for a modern Orthodox Israeli. Dr. Gal Meiri begins with his generous introduction of me but in an unusual detour, describing his tours of duty in Golani brigade (one of the elite units) in the first and second Lebanese Wars. I will return to this momentarily.

But I found as I write that I have multiple introductions. First to these doctors. I reminded them that neither Homer nor Virgil fought in the military wars they described. They were, however, the voices, the poets whose words are mere air until recited by the reader. The words emerge from the soldiers (and their families). I continued, "You soul healers are the poets who will speak the voices of the soldiers in battle."

Then I recounted a much more personal story, the story I told you, the reader, earlier in this book. My father, I continued, the aspiring high school engineering student, became a "guest" of the Nazi concentration camps, and after the Lodz ghetto fell, then moved to the Warsaw ghetto until it fell, until "graduating" from Auschwitz. The Nazis, I continued, and you, the reader recalls, put my father and his cohort on a death march out of Auschwitz. My father collapsed roadside.

Now, I leaned forward, turned to these physicians and psychologists who were involved in saving kidnapped Jews and protecting Israelis (Jewish and Arab). I spoke to them *b'gova eynaim*, eye-to-eye, with humility.

I continued,

You, the Israel army, are now doing what the American army soldier did for my father. You are saving hostage Jews and Israelis like that unknown American soldier did with my still breathing father. You pursue the enemy and are the soldiers saving Jews today. Please, let me help you with your tasks.

DOI: 10.4324/9781003618690-5

I wanted these officers to know that as they have gone to war to save Jewish hostages (and protect Israeli citizens from further attacks), so too some American had gone to war and freed him from Nazi slavery, even from death. So, I could barely express profound gratitude to these men.

I wanted to say more, but needed to hear their questions, their stories. Here, I will say a bit more to you.

In 2002, I chose to study Israeli soldiers of elite hand-to-hand combat units. I came about this idea thus. I had completed a study of 76 Americans followed from birth to 30, *Lives Across Time* with Henry Massie. Of the 76, about 14 were in our highest emotional-functioning category at the age of 30. All 14 had gone to elite Universities and were practicing professionals or academics. None of our American 76 ever was in the army. But I thought, in Israel, those who would be in the highest functioning categories would first go to army, then University. How would this Israeli cohort compare to our American group?

That was the question. I was funded by the International Psychoanalytic Association after an initial rejection: one panel member asked why I wasn't studying Palestinian "soldiers."[1] I responded, that I didn't speak Arabic, and likely they would not speak to me at all: I resubmitted the grant unchanged, which was funded.

Over the next few years, I made some two dozen flights to Israel, interviewing former soldiers who were turning 30, like our cohort.[2] But I also had the good fortune that the Israel army has a rating system for new soldiers, the KABA score, that gives something equivalent to our measures for overall robustness; in fact, the KABA is likely stronger, as it measures academic ability, physical fitness, as well as behavioral (emotional) strength. I chose to study only those who entered elite combat groups (excluding those in the air force or 8,200 (intelligence/computer programming)), because a second question I wanted to pursue was how these men handled face-to-face combat; how did this affect them?[3]

You are getting a sense of my detour here. This is a detour of time, backward in order to understand my need to come to Israel after October 7. To listen to soldiers.

I will tell you briefly of the results of this earlier study, *Reluctant Warriors, Israel Between Rome and Jerusalem*, then take an even longer detour before returning to today, to post October 7, to life in Hell and after.

I chose not only to study soldiers approaching 30 but also to those who had done their required service, became officers, but chose not to continue an army career. But no Israeli *really* leaves the army because of annual *miluim*, training and of course, call-up for wars. I stumbled into this awareness when I greeted a now-grizzled, exhausted physician colleague, a father of three, a man approaching 40, as he returned from his annual *miluim*. I welcomed him back. Bending his head to light a cigarette, he asked about the progress of my study. I mentioned that I had re-interviewed my guys because they had been called up to the Second Lebanese War. That I was interviewing guys who were not in *keva* had "finished" the army service. I realized my *faux pas* as the words slipped from my lips. He, gracious, glanced up silently from this cigarette, red-eyed, slump-shouldered, and I realized that he still, at 40, as a physician, he still served. Israel is a militarized but a *not* militant society. It is more Athens and reluctantly Sparta.

In short, I found that those Israelis who had highest *kaba* were recruited into the toughest "elite" units. They did "well" afterward—completing college in three years, some going on to get master's or doctoral degrees. One, for instance, who got a double bachelors in three years, was the COO of a start-up in another country, and a few years later became the CEO. I asked about his success. He responded, that after the army, business is no big deal. Another emphasized this closeness with fellow soldiers (he was in tanks, where being close *is* the nature of battle). Sardines. Or they would joke, "the toaster." Now, doing a postdoc in another country, he mentioned that if he ever needed his buddies, he just needed to call and say, "I need you." He wouldn't have to say why; they would just fly over. He was proud of his self-built apartment decor, attributing it to his "on-the-fly" innovations he learned to keep his tank in repair on the go.

The more difficult conclusion (difficult perhaps for American readers) was that these guys were different in character in a specific modality: greater maturity, more somber at times. And more focused on marriage and having children in contrast to our 30-year-old American subjects. One of my Israeli soldiers, a bright, handsome fellow now approaching 30, was worried: he said that he hadn't married yet. He had "played around" with Israeli girls. Now, he wanted to get serious, find a wife, have a family, and return to Kibbutz.

But, while writing the soldier book, like the slingshot use of gravity to send satellites further into space, I found myself flung further back in time. Bear with me.

I realized my debt to Roy Grinker, Sr., my first psychiatry chairman, with whom I never spent enough time. Grinker, then in his forties in WWII, volunteered for the US army and was sent to North Africa, into that maelstrom engineered by Rommel. In brief, Grinker (and Spiegel) designed the first successful field treatment for acute War Neurosis, that ailment described in WWI (then called shell shock) that often resulted in decades of suffering debility. Grinker pointed out that what we now call Acute Stress Disorder (ASD) or reaction can appear phenomenologically with various psychiatric "faces," including psychosis.[4] More significantly in his book, Grinker showed the first successful treatment of ASD: treat near the front, treat immediately, use short-acting barbiturate IV to induce a slight hypnotic state, and then ask, "What happened? Tell me what happened." The soldier would begin to recite with terrifying feelings what happened; some even leaped from the bed or gurney, crouching in fear as if carrying a weapon and pointing in the direction of "fire." Then, following symptom resolution in many cases, Grinker sent the soldiers back to their units (Grinker and Spiegel, 1979).[5] Some eight decades later, Z. Solomon used these three approaches: proximity in time place, hope, and return to the unit in her work in the Lebanese war. (This was portrayed in the movie *Dancing with Bashir*, which included Solomon.)

For *Reluctant Warrior*, I realized I was following in Grinker's footsteps. But, after October 7, now in my eighth decade and with Israel in the greatest threats to its existence since at least 1948, I felt, perhaps like Grinker, that I needed to be with my people to fight evil as best I could, as a physician, as a psychiatrist, as a psychoanalyst,[6] and as a *mensch*.

My people? My family *includes* the people of Israel. I rarely spoke about my background. One of my supervisors in Chicago pressed me about my father's experiences in Auschwitz; I said I wouldn't discuss this. A colleague in New York said that he was in a study group with Judith Kestenberg; all the others had interviewed a child of Concentration Camp survivors; could he interview me. I refused. I wanted to be known for what I did and said, not for my father's suffering. I felt that there was a voyeuristic quality to other requests; one Israeli therapist on the East Coast made a living interviewing and writing about children whose parents had been in concentration camp. Voyeurism. Janet Malcolm wrote sensitively, honestly about how biographical authors live off of people about whom they write; a form of parasitism. So, I felt about those who pried about my parents' experience. For this work in Israel, I needed to reveal my gratitude and connection with these officers.

Grinker. I recall well my first meeting him, being interviewed for a residency position. He was the penultimate interviewer. He greeted me at his door, my folder before his face and cigar smoke emitted as if from my file. He demanded gruffly, "Szajnberg? Why didn't you change the spelling of your last name?" I answered, even as he was turning away from me, expecting me to follow, "I've changed enough things in my life." He began chuckling through his cigar, the puffs arising like smoke rings. I realized later that Grinker accepted me based on that response (although my CV looked pretty good). I was accepted by Reese but turned them down, despite its history of being the most desirable residency in Chicago. It was because of my last interview. Dr. W. kept me waiting for some 20 minutes (I later learned he would do this with clinical meetings and others). He too had attended the University of Chicago and got both his MD and PhD there (in sleep studies, which I had toyed with). W. pointing his forefinger at me like some Uncle Sam, and said in his high-pitched voice, "I *want* you!" I knew then I would choose to go elsewhere.[7] I returned to Reese when the other residency program was turned upside down by a new director.

You see how long this backward-flung detour. Let's listen to these modern Homers and Virgils who carry the voices of soldiers in their minds, in their hearts.

Dr. A. begins. He has a soldier who works in *Zaka* (like search and rescue). On October 7th and thereafter, his responsibility was to enter Be'eri and other *yishuvim* to save those alive and gather up the dead bodies . . . and body parts—heads, limbs hacked off or blown to bits by grenades tossed into crowded bomb shelters.[8] He came to Dr. A. with a disturbing symptom. He recalls one young dead woman whom he tried to lift alone. Blood stained her bare legs; she'd been raped before death. Usually, two men carried a corpse; but there were too many dead, not enough colleagues. How to carry her alone? He raised her by her torso his hands beneath her hips, to port her limply, her arms and legs dangling, rape blood dripping down her legs, to the vehicle. When he returned home after months of service, he found that when he romantically embraced his wife in bed, the image and the feeling of this slain young woman leapt into his mind. "Please," he implored this physician, "please cleanse me of this image."

Dr. B. offered a soldier's recurrent nightmare since serving in Gaza:[9] his younger brother is dead, laying upon and suffocating him as he hears his young daughter's voice crying. Dr. B. also knows that this Orthodox soldier is a *ben ha'bachur*, "the chosen son" (the first-born son), which carries extra sense of responsibility. The doctor says to the dreamer that the dream may reflect his extra sense of responsibility, and this seems to mollify the soldier. Working with acute stress in a war setting doesn't afford us the time, the attitude to explore dreams and lives more fully. At times a "deep" (or "Kleinian") interpretation can be ventured, such as the dream reflects your ambivalence about your brother, how your brother may be smothering in your life; how your daughter's cries keep you alive. And we know from Freud (1900) that characters in dreams may be disguised—the "brother" may represent a compilation of others, even the soldier's self-smothering his own self; the daughter representing another. Or the crying alive daughter may represent the girls he saw slaughtered in the *Otef*; he brings them back to life in his nightmare/dream.[10] These are speculative and perhaps might have helped. But we are not going to second guess this physician at the front line and the relative relief his comment offered the soldier.

One example presented by a soldier from a very elite unit[11] is as follows. He and his three brothers all were qualified for this tough unit. But the army was reluctant to permit all four to serve in this very dangerous capacity. Nevertheless, the brothers were adamant and got the army to agree that they could serve in the unit, provided each brother was in a different team. The brother who approached me was speaking for his siblings: they were one of the first units to enter Be'eri[12] where there were dozens of corpses, some burned alive in cars; some beheaded; babies roasted in ovens; dead women with amputated breasts and blood streaming down their legs from multiple rapes.[13] Shortly after, they were sent to the coast north of the Gaza Strip to confront terrorists disembarking on the Israeli shore. The brothers and their units killed all the terrorists. Every one. But they came to me imploring that the sights of the slaughter at the *yishuv* remain seared into their mind, like branded cattle; not the danger of confronting the terrorists or the dead terrorists. How can they, these elite soldiers, relieve themselves of this vision?

Then there are the shades of adverse symptoms that are short of a diagnosis of ASD; even if not debilitating, one feels impaired, less than one's optimal self. Two officers from *Egoz* and *Shayetet* are now back in professional school after months of duty in Gaza. After talking for a while, they both admit that they are having difficulty concentrating on their professional studies, which they had been preparing for years before October 7. They find a kind of buzzing interruption in their concentration, distractions from the subject at hand. And when they walk down the streets of Tel Aviv, they find themselves scanning the second floors, the windows, and the balconies, with focused anxiety, scanning for snipers. Finally, another preoccupation is with the well-being of their men, even if they are not currently deployed in Gaza. One senior officer, now in the reserves, confessed, much to his wife's dismay, that he has two cell phones on his belt: one for his wife and family, the other for men in his unit. He told them that they could call him anytime for any reason, even if it were something personal. His wife then told me that this man's buddy from the army planned to build a weekend shack in a very remote area (Judeah). Her husband agreed immediately to build a shack next to his buddy, so he wouldn't be alone. Such are the connections among those in combat units in particular (Janowitz et al.).

Let's return to the matter of treating ASD, not just during war but within a war zone.

We will hear some seat-of-the-pants ideas that are tailored during war. Let's listen patiently, and respectfully, knowing that like Grinker's work, over time, some things will pan out, some not. War does not favor "controlled" studies in the standard sense. (When we submitted some of these interventions to professional journals, some insisted that we get informed consent from the soldiers, have control groups. War does not permit niceties.)

Yoni Elkins, a social worker is head of the medical team in the south for evacuated soldiers with psychic trauma. Trained in EMDR and a dedicated runner, Yoni developed the following approach with ASD. It involves jogging or running, requests to recall the episode, and working through it. His edited account is here:

First, sense, feel, taste, smell, and hear the setting of "treatment." A setting just outside the front, but rockets hit, explosions heard:

> The therapist comes to the soldier, to his unit, outdoors, sometimes in a military tent, sometimes on the base desert parking lot. Clouds of sand, dust blowing.

I arrive with the full military dress code including my rifle, so the soldier knows I'm not an outsider. Yet I try to look informal (given that I'm an officer). I apologize for changing my boots to running shoes that I always carry with me in my backpack; if I were to do this "training"[14] with military shoes at my age my feet won't last. This often breaks the ice. The noises, smells, and sites are those common to the military field, not built military bases that are further from the front.[15]

The principles of this acute stress reactions training (treatment) are as follows:

1. Brisk walk with the soldier asking him to tell the story of the traumatic episode in sequence. If he can't tell the chronological sequence, ask him for the scenes he remembers; later, reconstruct the chronological sequence together. The fast walk allows an energetic discharge . . . *and* the soldier slows when recounting the traumatic episode; the soldier disconnects from the here and now. The only interventions are "Then what happened?" or "Keep the walking pace."
2. Ask him to upload the first image he would like to process. Make sure it's one specific moment, a still image. Then, ask what feeling comes up and its body location.
3. Ask the soldier to take this feeling as a type of energy that he needs to *stay with and fuel him* for a set of runs. Ask him to run at an easy pace for about 50 meters, while concentrating on the image and the bodily sensation it evokes in him and to be with the feeling as much as possible. Ask the soldier if he prefers running alone or together. This both restores a sense of control and choice and also offers togetherness. Even if he chooses to run alone, he knows he can change his request. If you run together, the therapist runs at the same foot-stomping pace as the patient, but with a little more stomping than the patient in order to echo his steps and enhance the feeling of togetherness.
   When he finishes a set, ask what he noticed. Then encourage him to repeat the "run with the feelings." Continue with another set.
4. Usually symptom, improvement takes about five sets. The trauma event is described as more distant, and less overwhelming. At this stage, we ask him to give lighter words for this moment (such as "it's over"/"you can start digesting," etc.), and we go for another set this time of skipping instead of running.
6. If there is no improvement between sets explore one of three reasons: (a) the patient does not stay with the emotion enough (e.g., feels nauseated and does not give it space); (b) the emotion is a *reaction* emotion and not a source (*original*) emotion (e. g., anger or guilt instead of helplessness); and (c) the emotional flooding is related to foul smell.

If the reason is the first—feelings fade prematurely—encourage him to stay with the emotion. For instance, staying with nausea often means to the point of vomiting. With another two sets, the patient starts to vomit and feels as if he releases all the disgust that is trapped inside him.

If the reason is the second, "secondary versus primary emotions"—explain the difference between source (primary) emotions and response (secondary) emotions and help focus on the source emotion and go to another set.

Third, smell is a more primitive feeling, not an emotion of course.[16] Smell may respond to early intervention. We need further clinical research to release the flashback of the smell.

So far, I have personally treated dozens of soldiers in this way and also a significant number of military personnel who did this under my guidance (over 10 military personnel) testified that they had the same reactions. I also had the opportunity to do this intervention twice (two different soldiers) by telephone because they were too far away (e.g., in the North when I was in the South).

Case Examples:

One soldier had another *kaban* trying to calm him down, but it was clear he was in a full flashback, pacing back and forth repeating "I gotta get outta here. This isn't for me." He was rubbing his nose as if trying to get rid of the stink.

When I approached him, he appeared not to notice. I gave him a pat on the back and said, "I'll help you outta this" (very calmly but assertively). Then he looked at me. I said, "See that tree there? I'll race you to it. Trust me, it'll help." He bolted out and ran way past the tree that was about 20 meters away. He ran about 500 meters in full-blown sprint. When he finished he headed back to me while I ran toward him to catch up. He seemed able now to communicate. I told him who I am, and that I'm here to help him out. He said, "I want to go home, that's what I need." I suggested we first fix what he's going through, because home right this moment not only won't help but also will make it more difficult to get out of it. I suggested he try to let me help him and he agreed on the condition we discuss going home after. I agreed.

I asked him to join me on a quick walk (about 6 kph) while he described everything he just went through.

He didn't remember.

"Just say whatever you say, afterwards we'll make order out of it."

He shared the horrors of going into the border Israeli villages on October 8, and collecting all the bodies, parts, everything he saw, and the smell of burned flesh that won't leave him. I gave him some concentrated lavender oil fragrance that I had on me for this purpose. The smell calmed him.

After he finished telling the story, I repeated it to him making sure he agreed about the sequence and nothing else came to mind. When dissociated it was hard to remember the events chronologically. I used the Fragmented Traumatic Events Protocol procedure to build the narrative.

I asked what *moment* he would like to release from his system first.

He told me the moment he saw a baby beheaded by the terrorists and another baby shot in the face. I asked him what emotion comes up and he told me, disgust. I asked him where he felt it in his body. He told me: his belly, as if he would vomit.

I explained that this overwhelming physical sensation is energy, and I want him to use this energy to run to the tree and back. We did three sets. Then, he reported the image being farther away from him. When asked how disturbing or overwhelming it is for him now he reported "It isn't right now."

We did the same to two more points of disturbance, one of which was with the smell of burnt flesh from the bodies at *Kibbutz Be'eri*. Both symptoms dropped to zero on the ESR scale.

He searched the entire narrative and found no more points of disturbance. Then, I asked him for a positive statement maybe of growth for the event. He said, "Maybe I can handle it after all." We did another set of skipping instead of running and rethinking what he just went through. Skipping brings a more childish and lighter tone to the exercise.

Now, he was prepared to talk to his officer to return to action.

At two-week follow-up, he'd returned; he feels connected to the unit and his comrades; he has no post-traumatic symptoms. Feels good and meaningful in his job.

Case 2:

After this soldier's base got shelled, he felt very overwhelmed, agitated, loud sounds made him jump, and he's hyper-vigilant. He had trouble with sleep-onset for the last two nights.

I asked, "Tell me the story while we walk fast."

It's a war zone, so his officer cleared where we would walk, so we wouldn't get shot by friendly fire.

Thrice we ran as he told the story and identified a point of disturbance. His symptoms dissipated. On follow-up next day and week, he said all is good, he felt back to himself, and returned to his unit.

Most treatment settings are outdoors, in the field. Just two army dudes running off what one of them just went through. While therapeutic, it doesn't look so unusual to other soldiers.

In other cases, we jog/talked in a park when on break from the army, or back on his base between deployments, or in the *Sde Teiman* IDF base parking lot. But not indoors.

They all reported something very easygoing that allowed them to express what they felt physically and not only talking about it, which they felt was more overwhelming.

A third example was a soldier who was exposed to dead comrades in a fellow tank that was hit. The smell in the tank of burnt flesh and metal stuck to him and he couldn't sleep. I was called to see him in his camp about a week after the event. We did the walk with narrative and started processing the moment he entered the tank and the smell came to him, and he started to feel nauseous. I suggested to give it a place and during the second set he stopped because he needed to throw up, "What's wrong with throwing up?" I ask. "Trust your system to do what it needs to process the event." Halfway through the third set, he threw up and reported feeling much better and released. We did a few more sets to make sure event was cleared. We closed with a positive statement.

In many cases, when I first meet the soldier, he doesn't look like a combat soldier: he looks weak, beat, deflated, slumped-shouldered, often pale, and defeated. After an hour or two of this intervention, I notice they are taller, their color returns: they look tough again, as combat soldiers tend to look.

In my medical company, I treated about 50 soldiers and I was allowed to follow them closely weeks later. None had recurrence of the disturbing images after we reached zero flooding in processing.

Zen in a War Zone: How to Build It. (with *Oded Arbel, MD*)

Where to start with Dr. Arbel's story? From Homer on, the writer suggests starting *in media res*, in the midst of an act of tension: Petulant Achilles refusing to go to battle; Aeneus escaping burning Troy, his father astride his shoulders directing him, his son in one hand, his wife, trailing behind, soon to be murdered; Danté, in the middle of his life, in a darkened woods. But, in Jewish biblical tradition, one begins "In the beginning," literally, "*Bereshit*" when all was *tohu v'vohu*, "welter and waste and darkness over the deep" (Genesis I, I; R Alter). Before light was separated from darkness.

Start in *media res*? Ironically, October 7 is closest to Dr. Arbel's and Israel's "welter and waste and darkness over the deep." Both the middle of his life and a harsh beginning. Dr. Arbel's student, Orit, was murdered in her home that day, and also the son of his student Rauma, Lior, was butchered in *Be'eri*: the depths of Hell. And at dawn, when light was separated from darkness, Dr. Arbel, a psychiatrist and Zen student arose to take care of the soldiers who were to fight in Gaza.

Start at the beginning? This might be in 2002, when Dr. Arbel, already a physician, served as a reserve combat officer on a reconnaissance unit in the southern Hebron Hills (where now, a prestigious *yekev*, a wine-making vineyard sits).[17] His experience there moved him to train as a psychiatrist to serve as commander of the Combat Stress Reaction Team, serving in multiple Gazan conflicts before October 7. Something else led him to study Zen including a stay in Kyoto. All this he applied to October 7 and its aftermath.

Listen.

On October 7, before any military order, Drs. Arbel, Shai Neustadt, Roy Sage, and Ziv Sofer drove through the fog to the base south of Beersheva.

Nothing was clear. Faced with the sense of failure (of our army and government) helplessness, surprise, the overwhelming casualties including civilians and vulnerability and lack of protection, I asked myself, 'Is what was known and practiced still relevant? It was as if the sun had risen in the West . . .

The first evening, the lights were dimmed and we were confined to inner rooms after an alert about an explosive drone. A dear and veteran friend, a graceful therapist and commander arrived without uniform after his family fled their home in the Gaza Envelope. Another friend also in the unit had a son fighting the invaders. . . . One of my student's daughters was kidnapped to Gaza and her son murdered. My children saw their father, the doctor, leave with uniform and weapon in the midst of sirens . . . It was no longer clear what was a safe place. Even our previous treatment setting was invaded by Hamas . . .

. . . The tendency to collapse, threatened the treatment team.

I read Dr. Arbel's words as I sit in my almost silent consulting room in Palo Alto. Over the years, I have learned how to sound seal my office: special double-pane glass (with differential thickness of the glass to decrease transmitted resonance), staggered-studded walls, silicon seals on doors and windows, and stacks of books that mute internal noise. A room-size Aubusson rug and other Southwest American flat-weave rugs also soften the ambiance. Now, listen to war's waiting room.

The senses are assaulted: the explosions, the stink (of ammunition, of death, the vile scent of burnt flesh), the sight of helicopters or bullet-riddled private cars returning from the *Otef* (Envelope) piled with dead or injured civilians. One even *feels* the compressive impact of explosions. The instructions to protect oneself from a missile if one is outside or in a car are to leap from the car, drop face down, cover your head with your hands, cross your legs, and open your mouth. Why, why, why, and why? The car is an explosive device if it is hit; face down protects your vital organs; hands overhead is (as if) you protect your skull; legs crossed to "protect" your leg femoral arteries from being pierced by shrapnel; and mouth open so that percussive sonar impact won't rupture your lungs. This is the external "treatment" setting within which Dr. Arbel and colleagues are trying to construct a healing center.

Listen: how to maintain a clear mind?

I saw two challenges: first, treating soldiers whose young eyes saw far too much (for) what a soul is capable of containing. The second challenge was to protect the psyche, spirit and consciousness of the team . . . and myself from collapsing into secondary traumatization, reduction and erosion of compassion . . . to prevent exacerbation and chronicity of trauma . . . (it) is still unclear how to deal with (this) . . . horror stories, sights and smells can cause closure depression and loss of faith. . . . (How) to keep the heart and mind open . . . full of compassion.

"Compassion," the OED defines as, "Suffering together with another, participation in suffering; fellow-feeling, sympathy" (1340–1635). And "passion" from the Latin *pati* means suffering, referring initially to Christ's suffering and beginning in the sixteenth century to sexual passion. Hence, "compassion" literally translates as "with-suffering." How does one listen with the earlier concept of *lev shomeah*, a "listening heart," King Solomon's one request from God, without being disrupted by the soldier/patient's suffering? We will return to this but note here the distinction between sympathy (feel or pain *with*) versus the psychoanalytic use of empathy (feel or pain *into*), the latter suggesting an emotional resonance without being overtaken by the suffering and with a sense of reason, as Freud wrote in a letter to Marie Bonaparte (Baudry, 2025).

Dr. Arbel begins by repairing and cleansing the setting, as if it were a surgical suite. The "clinic" has broken doors, bullet-shattered windows, and the mundane Negev desert sand and dust that pervades every crevice. The first sight of blowing sand and mini-tornadoes of dust reminds us of "dust to dust" (and "ashes to ashes") in Auschwitz, in *Be'eri* (Genesis 3:19) to which we shall all return.

Dr. Arbel and his cohort began at 4:30 a.m. as he did in his Kyoto temple; anyone late to the Kyoto Zen center could not enter.

Dr. Arbel's "Zen" army center is where the staff ate, slept, held staff meetings and group meetings. Their cleansing not only served "hygiene . . . but also distinguished between night and day . . . changing the energy to . . . free (us) from the events of the past day and night. He adhered strictly to morning and evening meetings," an anchor of stability within "a reality . . . of chaos and uncertainty."

Of course, the staff was

> dedicated to internal changing . . . staff meeting was devoted to discussing the feelings, sensations and moods of team . . . unloading an accumulation of difficult stories, making our togetherness present. Clinical and operational consultations took place spontaneously and organically.

The latter reminds us of Redl's concept of field interview working with delinquent adolescents that Bettelheim elaborated on in working with younger children. Both were students of Aichhorn et al. (1964), whose work with Viennese street "delinquents" initiated a cohort of analysts for adolescents that included Anna Freud, Erikson, Blos (1964) (one of my supervisors), Ekstein (another of my supervisors), Redl, and Bettelheim (my mentor).

In the morning, after cleansing, after light breakfast, after unburdening the previous day's assault, "we went out for sports . . . frisbee, soccer or basketball . . . a joyful and beneficial tradition."

Only then was the team ready to treat soldiers in distress. We leave aside for now some accounts of their treatment—you have already read about some cases earlier—to turn to the end of the day.

In the evening, another staff meeting "with . . . chocolate cookies and drinks . . . and a shared activity . . . lectures, often a movie."

What movies? *Apocalypse Now* (which ends in Conrad's "the horror the horror"), *Halfon Hill Doesn't Answer*, *Catch-22*, *The Band's Visit*, *Avanti Popola, and Golda.*

This in the United States we might call a busman's holiday. One of my soldiers, married, with several children (2006) who was a commander, rescued his unit, of whom five were killed. For years, he watched *Full Metal Jacket* repeatedly, in the evening; but alone, always alone. Watching alone did *not* bring relief; rather elicited guilt, survival guilt, and guilt for having sent the men into this ambush.

But for Arbel's team, there was also karaoke and songs that "reminded us of beauty and friendship and love of the land." Love of the land is a common theme in Israel. It is, as Moses said, *Eretz Zavat Halav, Halav U'dvash*, "A land of milk and honey." It is also, as Naomi Shemer sang, *"haoketz v'hadvash"* of the "bee stinger and honey."

Here, Dr. Arbel turns to Zen concepts that helped him conceptualize and construct this "Zen" in hell center. *"Upaya"*—use material skillfully to benefit and heal; the "creative and wise way in which compassion flows." All the activities earlier were intended to bring blessing to the tormented world. He draws a parallel between the Buddha's instructions on meditation body posture, which should be like tuning a string instrument: too tight and it might break; too loose and it won't play well. For him, treatment is listening and tuning.

But then, Dr. Arbel returns us to the dilemma of being *both* a physician (per the Hippocratic oath *premium non nocere*,[18] "First do no harm") and a soldier, his rifle patting his thigh as he walked. Listen to Dr. Arbel's candor:

> how quickly that rifle returned to being part of my body and the automatic movement of searching for the weapon with a pat on the thigh returned, as if thirty years hadn't passed since service in the reconnaissance platoon. Strange to be Israeli. . . . Small as I am, how will I remain clear in the face of . . . conflicting commitments . . . incessant bombardment and attack . . . constant sounds of explosions . . . and "explosive" stories. . . . My team and I were exposed to . . . the heavy burden . . . to make decisions that would cost human lives . . . to return a soldier to combat . . . or determine he is unfit for combat . . . placing additional burden on his comrades in the unit, increasing the risk to them, especially if he is vital . . . like a medic or sniper. . . . Conflicting commitments . . . to the state and the army . . . (versus) to the individual suffering soldier.

Arbel appeals to the now-dead Zen practitioner/warrior, Manjushri to "come to our Camp to give guidance and direction; but he was probably busy."
Arbel explores the vagaries of "boundaries" in war.

> What are the boundaries of my compassion. The sounds of shells fired day and night from one side against the rockets and mortars fired from the other . . . My . . . typical "place" that was supposedly ethically comfortable . . . standing by the victims of the fighting—became less comfortable when I (was) aware of the enormous suffering . . . on the other side of the fence.

He continues, "such (military) actions cause mental scars and severe damage, called moral injury."

He turns for guidance to three Buddhist principles that offer refuge for support, comfort, and protection: (1) the "teacher" (Buddha), (2) the ideological/ethical that organizes the life path (Dharma), and (3) "the community of friends walking together on the path" (Sangha). He uses Buddhist terms, but in Hebrew we can use *Elohim* (or *Navi*-prophet such as Moses), *Torah* (teachings), and *Kehilla* (community).

He quotes Chogyam Trungpa who wrote the paradoxical "The Tender Heart of the Warrior" (2019).

if you open your heart to the . . . world, you feel tremendous sadness . . . For the warrior, this . . . gives birth to fearlessness . . . . You allow the world to touch your heart . . . share your heart with others.

Arbel returns us to his team, which kept their hearts open (again I refer to "*lev shomeah*") to terror, anxiety, horror, and sadness that knock (even pound) on the door of consciousness.

Arbel ends his story with dedications to all those whom he knew were killed or kidnapped. But his penultimate words are a prayer, even to us: "May all those whose souls and bodies were hurt by war find relief, joy and peace . . . live in times of love generosity, wisdom friendship kindness and peace." His words are inclusive, compassionate, as we would hope from a physician. Recall that the great biblical scholar Rambam (Maimonides) was also a physician (Szajnberg, 2013). Arbel follows in his footsteps.

Reader, take a breath before we turn to "moral injury." And its healing.

Shay (2002) describes moral injury as a sense of "betrayal": the impact of perpetrating, failing to prevent or witnessing acts transgressing core moral beliefs. It differs from ASD/PTSD, which results from terror and helplessness.[19]

The soldier experiences betrayal of what's (morally) *right* not only by leaders who permit/order unethical acts but also by betrayal of one's own ethics. For instance, witnessing civilian harm.

The symptoms include guilt, shame, and anger (often at self, leader, or society). With time, this can lead to isolation feeling morally tainted or misunderstood; self-destructive substance abuse, self-harm, risky acts; questioning the meaning of life and one's role and whether justice exists.

One of my students, a soldier in an elite unit, chose for his BA thesis to interview his fellow unit soldiers some five years after required duty. One fellow soldier pierced his heart. A hero, someone whom he respected, now chose to live alone in a caravan (a trailer) in a desolate area. Away from humans he preferred to be. No marriage, no children, no contact with humans; only goats and chickens. Occasionally, he ventured into a town to sell his meager produce or do handyman work. My student was crestfallen, felt this man's soul was lost, at least to society, even to himself. Moral injury.

Shay emphasized community's (particularly fellow soldiers)[20] therapeutic impact, rituals, and talking about experiences. Shay works to help the person realize that this was *not a personal failing*; this *is* war.

I was surprised not that the officers I met with, like Dr. Arbel, mentioned moral injury, but had not read Shay's work. Yet they could have written the book. One young officer[21] reminded me, "*am boneh tzava, boneh am,*" "nation builds army, builds nation." Each nation has its own culture which affects the nature of the army. In the 1990s, the IDF (Israel Defense Forces) enlisted Asa Kasher, a philosopher along with others to draft the Code of Ethics, ten values for every soldier, listed alphabetically (so that each value is given equal weight).[22]

Nearing the end of our meeting, after various challenging acute stress reactions were presented, came moral injury. They spoke of the following. Most soldiers live within an hour, perhaps two from the war zone. They are stationed in Gaza for two to three months, with brief home breaks, 24 or 48 hours. They are expected to seek, destroy, yes, kill Hamas combatants, and then return home to their families to embrace a father, a mother, a younger sibling, a wife, or child. One young soldier in an elite unit, *Duvedevan,*[23] described attending the birth of his first son. In the delivery room, his wife offered him his newborn son. Yet the soldier hesitated; thinking, "How can these blood-stained hands touch someone so pure?"[24]

Another officer described breaking into a terrorist's home, now emptied, as the terrorist had escaped. But on the wall was a photo of the murderer and his children. The soldier felt conflicted: how could he kill a father?[25]

One soldier was ordered to enter a known bomber's home after midnight and kill him. He and his unit enter ascend the stairs (a vulnerable setting) and he leads silently into the bedroom . . . to discover the man asleep next to his wife. He can't pull the trigger. He disobeys his order (and was punished severely for this) and leaves them asleep. Be clear, he couldn't shoot a man lying next to his wife.

Finally, a contrasting example, perhaps. A mother told me of her soldier son operating in the Judeah and Samaria area. He and his unit successfully arrest a terrorist, even as the children are screaming and pulling at the soldiers' pants, the wife wailing away. As the soldier leaves, he reaches into his pocket for his wrinkled shekels and leaves them all on the kitchen table, perhaps a week's worth of his paltry pay. The mother tells me this story with mixed feelings: proud of her son's good heart; aware that on October 7, this arrested terrorist left only death and horror on the tables.

There are many more such daily but non-mundane dilemmas that create internal conflict. The conflict is not because Asa Kasher wrote Ten Commandments of Ethics; rather, the conflict is internal from how each soldier was raised to respect life.

When I wrote my soldier book, *Reluctant Warriors*, I found, comparing the elite Israeli soldiers with the highest functioning American 30-year-olds, that the only clear difference was in a tone of maturity among the Israelis, a sober (and even somber in some) sense about life. An urgency to marry, have family, to both *oseh chaim*, "make a life," and to be serious about one's life. In every other metric, our American and Israeli young adults were similar: bright, emotionally solid, thoughtful, reflective, and good citizens. Perhaps, having to traverse the gap from late adolescence to young adulthood by navigating life and death, the Israelis take on the more serious, more sober tone.

When I discussed my *Reluctant Warrior* book with three medical students mentioned earlier, all of whom had just emerged from months in Gaza, they were puzzled by the title. They at first understood the title to imply that Israeli soldiers were reluctant to be soldiers. I was appalled at myself for the poor word choice.[26] These young men were not at all reluctant to fight after October 7. In fact, they called themselves, *lohamim*, "warriors."

I found myself backpedaling, shamefully. I meant that these soldiers (and them also) wanted to be first sons, lovers, fathers, brothers, doctors, teachers, and not soldiers. They were not reluctant to fight; rather reluctant to not be what is ingrained in their souls—good productive human beings. This explanation seemed to mollify these three fine physicians to be.

I close with an image. One of my guides/guards I've mentioned before, Ro'i ("my shepherd"). He was laconic, a fellow of few words. He was on "break" from his Golani unit in Gaza, moonlighting as a guard for visiting Americans. But I tell you two stories about him. In December, with rockets still flying from Gaza, our bus of volunteers was guarded by Ro'i. It took me two days to figure out that his gun was in his waistband, discreetly tucked away. I mentioned to him that my children were concerned about my safety. He asked to FaceTime them.

"I am Ro'i, which means shepherd," he began. "Your father will sit next to me on the bus. I will protect him and send him home to you." My sons' grins filled the screen.

But the second story is about what kind of commander he was, this silent fellow. After we were given a somewhat wordy tour of one of the Israeli bases, with its mock-ups of Gaza City and Khan Younis, it was already dark. Someone asked Ro'i how he prepared his unit to enter Gaza. He paused. Then said, "We train and we train and we train. Not much to say after that." Then he paused again. "Just before we crossed the border, I looked back at the few homes with lights twinkling in Israel." I told my men: "Look. It's for them we fight."

The psychiatric officers are both healers and Homers: listening with their hearts to the stories of the Odysseuses and the Aeneases. I retell them both to heal our soldiers and to bring some healing to this nation and understanding to the reader's hearing heart.

Notes

1 And officially they don't have an army or soldiers.

2 On budget, I flew mostly stopovers. I learned that US airlines fly into Heathrow, but out of Gatwick to Israel, requiring a madcap dash from airport to airport. On another more pleasant note, on a Milan stopover, I became enamored of a pair of suede, zippered, rubber-soled Lorenzo Banfi shoes, but passed because of price. These shoes haunted me through my Israel stay, so I nabbed them on the way back through Milan. I wear them now as I type, tips shiny from wear.

3 This is related to what Jonathan Shay called "moral injury" an issue raised by the current officers with whom I met.

4 In a recent update, Or Duek and colleagues published a study demonstrating that post-traumatic stress disorder can appear in some 600,000 symptomatic permutations (Duek et al.).

5 Janowitz and colleagues demonstrated the power of unit cohesion in WWII; Spencer (2022) has updated this in his recent book.

6 Unlike Grinker, I did not feel that some of my country's citizens had my back; at least not the vocal useful idiots supporting Hamas and their fellow travelers (murderers, rapists, butchers, barbarians).

7 Ironically, I started at the University of Illinois, which then fired its residency director, whom I respected, and appointed someone who had much to be humble about. I phoned Reese to return and they accepted me. This resulted in an unfortunate set of experiences that I won't detail here. Suffice it to say, my initial reaction to Dr. W was emotionally accurate. I should have stayed away. Grinker retired one year later, leading to a plummeting of the training program, which has now been closed for decades. The underground tunnel to the Medical Hospital, when it was being dug, was known as "Grinker's Gulch."

8 According to Orthodox Jewish tradition, all bits of flesh and body organs must be found and buried with the torso. This gruesome task means hunting for blown-apart flesh fragments, gathering them up, even with tweezers, I'm told.

9 "Serving in Gaza" often included fighting on October 7 in the Envelope Israeli *yishuvim* and collecting the dead and dismembered. Often it is the sights of the slaughter that were more traumatic to very experienced elite soldiers than any sights battling the enemy. I will give examples of this.

10 This would be a variation on Freud's example of the father who dreamt that his recently dead son was crying out to him in his dream: even for a moment, the wish in the dream is that the boy still lived.

11 For confidentiality, I am not naming which unit.

12 Again for confidentiality, I omit the specific place.

13 For a painful account of the actual barbaric acts by Hamas, read the suicide letter of the young man who hid as he saw his girlfriend beaten, raped from behind by multiple men, then turned over to be taunted, then shot to death (X, 8/25/24).

14 I thank Harold Kudler, MD of the US VA, who suggests the term training rather than treatment for soldiers. They are accustomed to training and "treatment" could be alienating.

15 But almost anywhere can be a front in Israel, given attacks from Hezbollah, Hamas, Houthis, and threats from Iran and Syria (NS Comment).

16 The Olfactory nerve is the first (of 12) cranial nerve that enters the brain through the cribriform process and the ventral cerebrum to form the olfactory bulb. It abuts some of the "emotional" loci of the brain such as the dorsomedial forebrain.

17 My high school buddy, Ed Salzburg, is the Yenan, chief winemaker, there.

18 My University of Chicago Medical School autopsy arena—icy cold (the better to preserve the cadavers), circular, raked seats above for observers, and a domed ceiling. Around the bottom edge of the dome was written "Primum non nocere."

When we did autopsies, I would glance upward and think, "Too late for this one." But, when a dear friend, Benson Ginsburg, was on faculty and had to pick an internist for himself, he researched it: he asked which doctor was most accurate at predicting what would be found at autopsy. That became his physician.

19 I cite again Shay's powerful two books on Vietnam veterans: *Achilles in Viet Nam* and *Odysseus in America*. Here, where the geography is so compressed when the war remains ongoing, our Achilles and Odysseus are both in "Vietnam" and America, as one of our discussants was asked about this (2010).

20 Fellow soldiers, as many felt that others, even loved ones, could not understand the horror.

21 Michael Matias is the student, an officer in the IDF, who taught me this.

22 Only the first principle is not alphabetical: (1) devotion to mission and drive for victory. The remaining nine are (2) responsibility, (3) integrity, (4) setting a personal example, (5) human life's value, (6) purity of arms (doing the best to not harm non-combatants), (7) professionalism, (8) discipline, (9) comradeship, and (10) mission.

23 Duvedevan means "cherry." His family was of Middle Eastern origin, so he had the coloring and features of his parents' home of origin—let us say Iraq, or Syria. He spoke Arabic and had practiced the Palestinian accent and dialect. His job during the day was, to sit in West Bank cafes, in Tulquarm or Jenin, play Shesh Besh or drink syrupy Finjan coffee with hel and listen. Listen for upcoming planned attacks against Jews. At night, he and his unit would enter the prospective terrorist's home to either kidnap or kill him.

24 Remember that King David was denied the privilege to build the First Temple, as he had too much blood on his hands. If we are kind, we might think that David felt too much blood on his hands to build the Holy Temple, as did our soldier. His son Solomon was given that honor.

25 Yet we also recall how many of the sadistic, murderous SS officers were described as loving fathers. Supposedly.

26 I could not find a good translation for "reluctant" in Hebrew; "Meha'ssessim," is hesitant, which has a different meaning.

Reference

Aichhorn, A., Fleischmann, O., Kramer, P., & Ross, H. 1964. *Delinquency and Child Guidance: Selected Papers*, Eds. Otto Fleischmann, Paul Kramer, & Helen Ross. International Universities Press.

Baudry, F. 2025. *Collected Papers*. IPBooks.

Blos, P. 1964. *On Adolescence: A Psychoanalytic Interpretation* (1st Free Press Paperback ed.). Free Press.

Grinker, R. R., & Spiegel, J. P. 1979. *Men Under Stress: Reissued with a New Pref* (Reprint of the 1963 ed.). New York: Irvington.

Shay, J. 2002. *Achilles in Vietnam: Combat Trauma and the Undoing of Character*. Scribners.

Shay, J., McCain, J., Cleland, M., & McCain, J. 2003. *Odysseus in America: Combat Trauma and the Trials of Homecoming*. Scribners.

Spencer, J. 2022. *Understanding Urban Warfare*. Howgate Publishing.

Szajnberg, N. M. 2013. *Sheba and Solomon's Return: Ethiopian Children in Israel*. CreateSpace Independent Publishing Platform.

Trungpa, C. 2019. *Shambhala: The Sacred Path of the Warrior*, Ed. C. R. Gimian. Shambhala Publications, Inc.

5 Parents, Families, and Community

In this chapter, we shift to parents, families, and community. "Community" among the *Otef yishuvim*, whether kibbutzim or moshavim, has a different tone or meaning than Americans may be accustomed to, more *Gemeinschaft* (a group bound by affiliative, affectionate bonds) than *Gesellschaft* (a group based on contractual, mutual consent). Max Weber puts these on a continuum, and we know that there is tension between the two states of community.[1]

Dr. S has not been able to function as a physician since October 7. She goes through the motions with some of her older patients but is unable to take on new ones. We later recognize that she can deal with life before October 7th, not life after.

Her *yishuv*, *Netiv Ha'asara*, was hard hit on October 7. Her neighbors across the road were slaughtered, and friends remain kidnapped. On October 6, she lived in a small house with her husband and two children; next door were her in-laws of whom she was fond, and the next door over, her unmarried brother-in-law. She joked that the three houses were like an extended Bedouin family, a tribe (*shevet* in Hebrew) living comfortably together. Her husband was born on this *yishuv* and her children, a daughter, and son, marveled in his memories of growing up here. She and her extended family were "leftists" who dedicated one day weekly to drive Gazans for medical care to Beersheva, Soroka Hospital, wait for the day, then drive them back. She looked forward to living in peace with them.

This has been shattered. She cites a neighbor, former "peacenik," cited earlier in this book, who said that all he wanted to see in Gaza now were flattened potato fields to the Sea. And perhaps beyond.

Listen to her account of that dreadful day (and night). They hid in the *ma'amad* of the house for some 32 hours. Thirty-two hours, she repeats. After some time, the phone's batteries ran out, so her husband crawled out to the car to recharge them. He didn't say what he saw as he crawled across the porch; she discovered later. When she emerged, she saw the porch bedecked with one of the large paraglider chutes that the terrorists had used to fly in with motorcycles suspended. Momentarily, she thought he had recently landed but learned later that was during the first hours of the attack. She could trace his trail of death, across the road at the bullet-riddled house, the

DOI: 10.4324/9781003618690-6

torched people. For some reason, he had skipped her in-laws. And her house, she added, as if realizing it consciously for the first time.

Initially, her family and in-laws and brother-in-law were evacuated to a gracious sea-front hotel in Tel Aviv, albeit in separate hotels. People, particularly Americans, were overly generous with gifts. She thought her children were getting spoiled with boxes, wrappings, and toys strewn about (although a California Noserider Surfboard became the keel for one son's new life). They decided to rent a place a few blocks from the Mediterranean, and one of her sons introduced himself to surfing, now his preoccupation; almost daily after school, he grabs his board and "hangs five." She admits, reluctantly, that the education for her children is higher quality in Tel Aviv. Her daughter is in a premier basketball league. Yet her children want to return "home." But her husband, Kibbutz born and bred, won't go back. Refuses. She believes it is not only out of concern for the children's safety but also, the memories, the stench of death, and burnt flesh.

She? She misses her *yishuv*, the little house. She will do as her husband wishes, but even the kids ask when they can return. Her in-laws have already moved back; they insist that they are too old to be frightened of terrorists. Her brother-in-law lives elsewhere in Tel Aviv. She misses her tribe.

As we talked, she came up with two insights. First that they could go back to the home (not just a house) for weekends, of course for the longer holidays. They could pretend they are wealthy Tel Avivniks with a "cottage" in the country. She thinks her husband would agree with that. Perhaps, she decided, they will renew the Tel Aviv lease for another year and visit the Kibbutz; she will use the "excuse" that the kids miss their grandparents.

I responded that it sounded as if a part of her soul had been kidnapped, is being held hostage; the terrorists controlled the physical lives of those who remained kidnapped. But she should not cede her soul to the terrorists; this would be an additional victory for them.

She lit up at this second idea that a part of her soul, yes, a part, felt as if it had been kidnapped, chained and blindfolded, and enslaved. She would demand that back. She knew her soul could never be the same, but it could become whole. She lifted her hand, saying, that she realized now that she needed to return to treatment; her old therapist had died, but would I recommend someone? She made that connection and began repairing her life and returning to her physicianly duties.

This idea of soul-kidnapping, being held hostage, proved useful to others. It is related to "soul murder" (Shengold, 1991)[2] in abused young children who remain welded to their abusers, never free. (It is radically different than the Stockholm syndrome; it is *not at all* identification with the aggressor. Not at all.)

Dr. Or Duek is a young, albeit respected researcher in PTSD. He post-docked at Yale, but as usual for many Israelis learned his expertise via being in the

IDF well before then. He lives in *Bror Hayal*, a small *yishuv* with history eons old; when Jerusalem was felled by the Romans in 70 CE, surviving members were hidden in *Bror Hayal* and neighboring communities. Now, history had been reversed; *Bror Hayal* was evacuated, although he and some members have begun to return.

We met over Macchiatos in University's Aroma cafe, delayed by an elderly security guard's shenanigans at the University gate. I was interested in his work at Yale, where they experimented with Ketamine-induced PTSD treatment at the VA. Ironically, one of my old colleagues, Natti Laor, a world expert in trauma particularly with children, had worked at this same VA. Or explained the rationale behind Ketamine and PTSD: the idea is to "arouse" some of the stored and "forgotten" memories of the initial war traumata. Once trauma memories are aroused, recalled, and so the researchers theorized, the PTSD vet could sort them out with guidance and resolve them. As usual, theory far out-paced the results. I mentioned, however, that this reminded me of Grinker and Spiegel's (Flarsheim, 1994) innovative barbiturate-facilitated treatment of ASD in the North African WWII arena. Or quickly found Grinker's book on his phone and I was certain would be reading it shortly.

From his postdoc, Or had written what will become a classical paper on the over 600,000 symptomatic presentations of PTSD. This, I told him, also reminded me of Grinker's observation in the North African WWII arena, that "War Neurosis"[3] can present with very varied clinical pictures, ranging from florid "psychosis" to catatonia.

However, when he discussed a currently hospitalized soldier, Or was not interested in Ketamine-induced recall; he relied on good clinical listening, patience, and focus. His thoughtful compassion changed the tone of our barely touched macchiatos. I filed this for my upcoming meeting with the army mental health team in a few days.

Then, we turned to his home, *Bror Hayal* ("Soldier Selection") which had been attacked by Hamas and then evacuated. But, history, history, layers of history. When the Romans sacked Jerusalem in 70 CE, Rabbi Yochanan Ben Zakai established a *yeshiva* here, a refuge for the survivors of the Romans (also, in the better-known Yavneh and nearby Nir Am). The *yishuv* tradition was to light a candle at the gate for a newborn child. Then, more history. In 1947, the ancient town was settled overnight (in "stockade and wall"[4] rapidity) by Israelis and became a magnet for Brazilian Jews. They were attacked by local Arabs the next day. Now, ironically, the one-time refuge for evacuated Jerusalemites was now evacuated.

Or was now moving back with his wife and two sons, but not all members were moving back; some insisted they would never move back; others asked for more time. A tense matrix hovered within the community of about a thousand; this tension was complicated by mourning for those who would not return, were slaughtered, or kidnapped. There is a ripping, shredding of the community fabric.

Bror hayal was contending with the government about sending the children back to the same elementary school that still bore bullet holes in the walls, even as the shattered windows had been repaired. This school served several surrounding *yishuvim*; children were bussed in. Some parents insisted that a new school be built and that sending the children back to the old one, even if rehabilitated, would be too disturbing. The government refused to pay for a new school. Then, Or, drawing on the small cafe table with his fingertips, described the plans for building the new bus station for the children to go from *Bror Hayal* to the school. I recalled as he drew—his fingertip on the café table—the new children's center being completed at Kibbutz Erez: how the old children's center metal roof had been pierced by missiles, so the new one was built like a bunker: double concrete walls; few and high clerestory windows; reinforced roof—and how this ran against the grain of the Kibbutz parents who wanted to raise their children open to the land. Now, Or was detailing how there would be a protected corridor from their children's center to the protected bus waiting area. But there were moments of vulnerability between the waiting area and the bus; there were also openings along the corridor vulnerable to bullets, even rockets. One has but minutes to get the children off the bus to a shelter (and no shelter *en route*; hence off the bus and lying face down, hands covering head, legs crossed, mouth open, at the roadside). I palpably felt his concerns. A parent shouldn't have to be worried their children will be killed or injured by terrorists on the way to or from school . . . or ever. October 7 changed his thinking. I noticed the trajectories of our conversations from more intellectual concerns about PTSD or ASD, to concern about his children's well-being. I remember my guide Elhanon, living in a small town in the Center of Israel: a peaceful, tall willowy intellectual, after October 7, he fixed the rusty locks on his house and gate, replaced the deteriorating fence, and packed a gun when at home.

Or told me of their evacuation and their experiences in the hotel specifically. The hotel was in Tel Aviv,[5] luxurious. But they left after a few weeks because of how disruptive the teens of the various *yishuvim* had become. They were getting drunk, likely using drugs, misbehaving. None of this was familiar to him from living in his *yishuv* over the years. Or and family moved to a rental, and more recently back to *Bror Hayal*.

I asked others from different *yishuvim* about the experiences, specifically of the teens that Or described. I compare this to an account from the only Orthodox *Yishuv*, *Alumim*, along the *Otef*. Ironically, I learned much from an officer I met two decades ago for my soldier book, Amitai Porat, who lives on Kibbutz Kfar Etzion in the . . . what shall we call it . . . ancient *Yehuda* region or called "West Bank" by others. I spent a Shabbat there and was peppered with observations, including how this Kibbutz was possibly one of the safest areas in the country now.

For Amitai, I beg your patience for a historical digression. His father was Chanan Porat, once a member of Knesset, a "right winger," Orthodox. Chanan was fatter of 13 (one was adopted, but for Chanan, also orphaned, there was no difference). At celebrations—weddings, bar or bat mitzvoth, Purim—all of some five foot-four balding Chanan would hop onto a table and dance and sing joyously. Even those who differed from his rightish stance adored him.

Chanan too was orphaned by the rifles of the Jordanian army. His father was one of the 156 members of the Kfar Etzion Kibbutz who were captured by and surrendered to the Jordanians in 1948; then, lined up against a wall and murdered.[6] Chanan grew up in Jerusalem, able to see the iconic Oak tree that crowned his father's former Kibbutz. In 1967, 20-year-old Chanan was among those who liberated the Western Wall in Jerusalem. Afterward, he and a fellow Etzion orphan hopped into a Jeep, drove to their Kibbutz, liberated it from the Jordanian army. . . . Then, they called their officer for permission to liberate the Kibbutz.

This is Amitai's patrilineal background. When I taught at the Hebrew University (2007–10), Amitai was the *mazkir* (literally, Secretary, but more like the manager) of his Kibbutz. I watched it grow and thrive, including his building a (controversial) set of homes for Orthodox residents who were deciding whether to become Kibbutz members. The turkey farm became a high-tech center, clicking replaced clucking. I often spent Shabbat there as a guest of my close college buddy, Myron Joshua, and always felt warmly welcomed, and enjoyed both the sense of calm and the thriving children.

Now, Amitai was working outside the Kibbutz as the manager for Kibbutz *Alumim*, one of the few Orthodox kibbutzim in the *Otef*. Some kibbutzim have decided to hire "outside" managers, avoiding the pitfalls of having a fellow member and many of the travails associated with having a Kibbutz member rotate through the position.

Leaving morning Shabbat service, in the scrum of the outside courtyard, I asked Amitai about how *Alumim* members had reacted to the aftermath of October 7, more specifically, the teens. He listened to what I had learned from Or and others. And as usual, reflected quietly before answering. Yes, he noticed some "delinquency," such as some teens not following the rules of Shabbat. But no drugs and alcohol and certainly nothing that would be considered "delinquent" outside of the falling-off of religion. He reflected a moment longer. He observed that prior to October 7, the teens of Alumim had lived in their *yeshiva* where they studied. Living away from home was not a break from their peer community. Perhaps the *yeshiva* matrix immunized from more delinquent acts. And he saw that returning to the Kibbutz would resolve the issue of Shabbat, as the teens would be back in their milieu. A tone of optimism about the return that was unusual among the others returning to the *Otef*.

A pause before I continue with our last *yishuv* in the *Otef*. An intermission to talk about the Ethiopian community in Kiryat Malachi. For, how could I not describe the experiences of my former research assistant of two decades, Zahava and her five children, *all* now serving in the IDF, four in Gaza? My book on Ethiopian children in Israel (*Sheba and Solomon's Return*) is based on my work in Kiryat Malachi, at Bet Tzipora, the Ethiopian after-school program funded by Elie Wiesel, named after his sister, murdered in Auschwitz.

Zahava arrived in Israel and married with one child from Ethiopia. Like most of our mothers, she attended school there until about third or fourth grade. In Kiryat Malachi (a town founded by Moroccan immigrants who then resented the influx of Ethiopians), she was pregnant with quadruplets. The doctor recommended removing some so that the others would be more viable. She refused and gave birth to three boys and a girl. Her husband quit his job to help with the kids; then he didn't. He left to live with his mother; Zahava was on her own but with the help of Bet Tzipora community. He died some years back.

The quadruplets were six when I began my study of six-year-olds. Because some of the boys needed extra help in the Bet Tzipora after-school program, Zahava volunteered to be an assistant. Over the years, she completed her education in Hebrew and is now teaching in both the public school and Bet Tzipora. Kiryat Malachi is perhaps 10–15 minutes northeast of the *Otef* communities; it was not breached. But the new principal (who assumed his job in September and then was drafted in October for Gaza) asked for my help. When the children heard the very frequent "red" alarm of incoming rockets, they cried—not out of fear for themselves but fear for their father, uncle, older brother, or sister in the army, in Gaza, often, if not in the North.

Zahava's oldest son is in *Tzanchanim* (paratroopers); a recent computer engineer graduate, the war interrupted his job search. When I visited her home, it was when he was on leave for a day or so. I noticed his body armor standing on a table; it was more like a saddle. I lifted it, a heft of perhaps 40–50 pounds. His younger three brothers are now deployed in Gaza; his sister is in the army in Hebron, also not such a peaceful setting for Israeli soldiers. But Zahava is relieved that her daughter is in Hebron, at least. Like many Ethiopian Jews, Zahava adds some blessing to God after speaking about each child. She herself is soldiering on; teaching the high school students by day, Bet Tzipora in after school; cooking and cleaning her new apartment for the kids, who still live with her. This is the first home she has ever owned, and it is dear to her that she has a home of her own for her adult children.

Zahava manages as she does with four kids in Gaza and one more safely in Hebron, in part not only because of an inner strength but also because of the Bet Tzipora community. *Gemeinschaft*. She is highly regarded at the school. What can one say to a mother of five all of whom are in the army, four in Gaza?

I'll finish this "tour" back on the *Otef*. Sh., a psychologist is returning to Kibbutz Erez, now "infamous" for being at the Erez crossing into (and from Gaza north).

Sh. is an academician. Before October 7, she drove some two hours to her University several days a week. Now, she spends more time at home, as she and other Kibbutz members are returning. She gave us a tour of the Kibbutz, at first wanting us to admire the new women's center, but later to see the old children's center destroyed by missiles, the new children's center described earlier, the communal eating hall and the Amish Australians who were donating several months there helping to rebuild the Kibbutz. Only at the end and only at my host's insistent request did we ascend the ridge overlooking Erez Crossing: the road, that artery of death, that ran through the *yishuv* below us, *Netiv Ha'asara*, Dr. S's *yishuv*, where many were slaughtered.[7]

I'll get to the view from the Kibbutz Erez ridge of the road of death from Gaza through *Netiv Ha'asara*. But I'll start with what I heard about the state of this *yishuv*.

Not all plan to return, Sh. said. She and her two children and husband have just returned (this is in July 2024). Sh. has been overseeing the new women's center construction, so she has been visiting often. She tells us that above her home's entrance are two bullet holes. She wanted to have those repaired before her kids saw them. But she didn't have time and hoped they wouldn't notice. Of course they did. When we walked by her house, she pointed out the bullet holes well above the doorsill. I suggested she get a sturdy stepladder and some colorful paint or indelible markers and have both kids paint decorations around the pockmarks. Funny characters like from the Moomen family or Peanuts or some fairy tale, perhaps Alladin and his Robin Williams' bluish genie.

Sh. spent much time showing us the still-empty women's center. She explained that funding came about when a wealthy American donor asked her what the Kibbutz needed most; Sh., a staunch feminist, said a women's center: a large central hall with movable walls and a yoga room and meditation and massage rooms. Their activities for women only sounded lovely. Dr. M and I looked at each other hesitantly—perhaps both of us thinking of the men who had died from this Kibbutz, or men currently in Gaza—then asked softly, "What about the men.?"

Sh. appeared stumped. Well, men are not allowed. Well, they have a pub some Tuesday nights. We asked, "Do the men on this Kibbutz like to congregate at the pub like in Ireland or England."

"Not really, but they can if they choose."

What seemed missing here was any discussion among the returning community of what is their hierarchy of needs. Of course, a women's center is lovely. But what of the men, at least those who hadn't been killed or kidnapped. What about a communal center for families? Maybe even a family evening weekly in this tasteful center. These are questions that could have been discussed by the returning community before building began.

But on to the new children's center being completed. I've mentioned earlier that the old one was now useless since its reinforced metal roof did not withstand missiles. Men were finishing the new, highly reinforced double walls (reminiscent of Masada, I found myself remembering, where the Jews stored dried food to withstand the Roman siege). We passed by the modestly dressed Amish workers. Deeply moving to have them here, but I found myself wondering if it would be reparative to have the returning residents working alongside me. Some father from another town, perhaps Ashkelon, had built small picnic tables with his son for the children.

Then the storied ascent. As we trudged up, Sh. and Dr. Meiri explained that each *yishuv* has its own volunteer guard. Erez got a heads-up to send its men to the ridge armed. The ridge is a slight arc. Later we could easily see the Erez crossing to our left with a high-flying taut-snapping Israeli flag. Directly in front and stretching to our right is *Netiv Ha'asra*, where much carnage was done by invading marauders. Sh. pointed to the narrow straight ribbon of road through Erez crossing and thrusting its way through *Netiv Ha'asara*. She pointed to the sky, silently as first, as if transfixed. Then, she reminded us that the invaders also glided in on paraglider with revved motorcycles suspended beneath. Whereas *Netiv Ha'asara* members were told to stay in their shelters (for better protection from missiles), the *Kibbutz Erez* guards were lying prone here and firing at the invaders. I looked again, as Sh. pointed out a white "tender" (a small four by four open back truck) lifting a faint trail of dust from east to west. I could barely make out the truck and marveled at the marksmanship of the Erez riflemen to hit targets at this distance. Not enough to protect the *yishuv* later.

We returned to the *chadar ochel*, the communal dining room, now beginning to fill with the Amish workers and others for lunch. The Kibbutz is too small to have its own kitchen, so food is packaged and shipped in.

We digressed a bit, as Sh. began to talk about her own research and I connected it with work on emotions by my friend and colleague, Paul Ekman. How lovely it will be to bring this other community—one of inquiry, of discovery—back to a life of higher civilization when we can discuss intellectual matters and less so tragedy and horror, from which they will recover.

For now, our task is to how to help. I venture some suggestions later.

Let's remember Aristotle on the optimal size of a city-state (*The Politics*, 1932). It should be self-sufficient, governable (citizens know each other, feel a sense of community) interact directly, large enough to defend itself (yet not have an unwieldy military) and have cultural, educational, and economic advantages. Or, we can turn to the book of the Bible, in which Moses designs legislative, judicial, and military roles within each of the 12 tribes for the descendants of the 600,000 Jews who left Egypt and wandered 40 years in the desert. Roughly speaking, this would be each tribe with some 50,000 men and their families.

The *yishuvim* I describe earlier are each some few thousand souls, some smaller in the hundreds.[8] If we return to Tonnies'/Weber's 1966; Weber and Tribe, 2019) ideas of the tension between *Gemeinschaft* and *Gesellschaft*, we get a sense of how *Gemeinschaft*, the felt bonds, the emotional connections, among the *yishuv* members are stronger than one might find in cities, even in some neighborhoods.[9] As for *Gesellschaft*, the kibbutzim had generally organized around agriculture (many were mainstays in this Desert, of agricultural produce in the Negev). Some had developed specialties, such as honey production, or now, high-tech innovation, or like Or and Sh, many worked outside the Kibbutz in academia.

Protection? Military. October 7 was a face slap for them, almost all of whom had served in the military and were in reserves. Yes, most had local civil defense guards from the members, but few bore arms. In one Kibbutz, many were saved by the actions of a young 20-some-year-old woman. She realized early on something was very wrong. She told the maintenance engineer to cut electricity so that the Kibbutz electric gate could not be opened. Then, she ran to the "armory" to hand out rifles and guns to the members who ran to her call. In a talk by a veteran Kibbutz *Re'em* member, he emphasized the new attitude. Yes, they would advocate from the central government for better irrigation, education, and so on. But, for local security, they were now bearing arms, as was evident from the gun in his holster. In another farm at the Egyptian border, the friendly, charming, engaging Orthodox father of several, openly bore his gun at his belt. In the past, he did this to warn off smugglers across the Egyptian border; today, it bore heavier intent. These men considered themselves the point of the spear for their families, their communities, at least until the IDF responds.

––––––––

"(October Seven) changes not just the future, but (also) the past . . . a realization that things will never be the same . . . and not what we thought they were before" (*Israel Alone*, Bernard-Henri Lévy, 2024).

And when the heart is silent,
The soul screams . . .
When the heart cries/
Time stands still.
     (Grinspan et al., 2000)

"Give me a listening heart" (King Solomon's request of God).

How to write about repair, rebuilding when the war continues, when parents fear for their soldier children in Gaza, near Lebanon and also for their little children, as seven countries—but really driven by voracious Iran (and the Bank of Qatar)—vow to *and* try to erase Jews?

My host, Gal Meiri tells of his "regular" (required) service in Golani in the first Lebanese War: the horrors seen; the decisions made of life and death. Later as a physician and (not quite former) infantry, he was asked to provide psychiatric care for soldiers. At first, he demurred, preferring to be hands-on with his men, and tend to their overt wounds. Later, seeing the suffering of hidden wounds, he switched to becoming the psychiatrist. But even then, even in the second Lebanese War (2006), he is hands-on. Stationed at the border, his unit of physicians and others were responsible for the MD's who were in Lebanon and then for the more serious injuries, to triage, to treat, and if need be, to ship out rapidly.

I've told you how years ago, when the early helicopter emergency program began at Soroka, Dr. Meiri, upon hearing the whomp-whomp of arrival, excitedly stepped to the window to watch the landings. Today, not so. Today, with the almost everyday arrival of helicopters from Gaza, he knows that this means terrible casualties aboard and if casualties aboard, then likely soldier fatalities in Gaza. His close friend and former student, once an ENT surgeon, Y. was coptered in with a shrapnel head wound; he was unrecognizable to his fellow physicians in the ER. Life saved, Y. is now in lengthy rehab, hoping to be able to speak again.

Now, Dr. Meiri can't bear to look at the arrivals, barely to hear. His son was deployed in Gaza and as I write, is preparing to deploy again. And his other son? Called to duty in the flaming north. (This was before the "pager" project that deflated Hezbollah.) Just north of where Dr. Meiri's parents and siblings live. How is he, he asks, to attend to the psychic ailments of patients when his mind is divided? And yet, I observed, he does.

A story from Tulquarm, that West Bank rat's nest of suicide bombers. Dr. Meiri's unit was embattled with terrorists and wounded one severely. When his men brought the terrorist out on a stretcher, Dr. Meiri performed what was second nature as a physician—he stabilized the wounded terrorist, then shipped him to the nearest Israeli hospital. He confesses that, unlike his usual practice, he did not inquire afterward of this fellow's outcome.[10] This perhaps is the other side of moral injury: when the enemy is armed, attack; when wounded, heal. But ambivalence, normative ambivalence remains. We remember Sinwar, Hamas's Gaza leader, was both diagnosed and cured of a brain tumor when he was an Israeli prisoner; and we know how Sinwar repaid.

So let us attend to the parents, the families, the communities, and think about how to rebuild even as this war for existence rages.

I return to my earlier comments on *Sinat Chinam*, the "free-floating" hatred of brother for brother, citizen for citizen. The inner wars. As Naftali Bennett cautioned, if this continues unabated, we will suffer as did the Jews of the Second Temple. Internally vulnerable because of fractious infighting, the Romans destroyed Jerusalem, stole the Holy Tablets, ravaged the country, and renamed the Jews as "Palestinians." Iran, perhaps even Erdogan's Turkey, is today's Rome, including as Empire-driven colonialists.[11] And the Jews of Israel may be too much like the Jews of the Second Temple.

Further, as Bernard-Henri Lévy warns, October 7 changed our perception of the past. Many, but *many* Israelis (and for sure Westerners), had this belief that if economic benefits and freedom were offered to the local Arabs, they would desire or at least live in peace. But October 7 unveiled unvarnished hatred, blood lust—lust in the sense of *passionate* desire for death—not only of Jews of course but also of fellow Arabs in both Gaza and the "West Bank." Trust is eroded, if not lost. Even the Bedouins I visited in Rahat fear that they too, despite being grateful to Israel (to some degree, barring envy), despite being targeted by Hamas, they have lost the trust of Israeli Jews. My college buddy, Myron, who lives on Kibbutz Kfar Etzion, is concerned that his Kibbutz can no longer hire local Arabs; and that those Arabs who have agricultural fields bordering Jewish settlements are restricted from working their fields within some yards of the Jewish areas. After all, the reasoning goes, Hamas had details of each Jewish settlement, details they likely gleaned from interrogating the Gazans who had been working on these settlements. How to repair (the word "heal" may be too hopeful) this gash in the local Arab-Jewish social fabric is a greater question and beyond this chapter.

Here, we must be humbler about what we can do for those in the *Otef* and neighboring communities. The ideas (suggestions) below for family, for community, are seeds that can be sown on an earth that is not episodically ripped up by *Sinat Chinam* or its seedlings uprooted by the stranger in a strange land, as the Jews were in Egypt and as they are commanded to treat respectfully the non-Jews within their midst. On the other hand, as a psychoanalyst, I do find that building from within (the individual, the family, and the community) can contribute to mutual regard that ameliorates *Sinat Chinam:*[12] if one feels secure about one's identity (internally), one can judge external reality more accurately, who is a true enemy.

I must add my response to Robert Alter's personal and thoughtful critique of my term *Sinat Chinam* for the civil unrest in Israel prior to October 7. Reading an early version of this manuscript, Alter argued that this wasn't *"chinam,"* *free-floating.* Rather, he insisted the government's suggested changes to rebalance the Supreme Court, which had aggrandized greater power in the 1990s, was a legitimate reason for the anti-government demonstrations. Not *chinam* at all, Alter insists.

I wrote that version and received his thoughtful critique around Hannukah, the holiday which celebrates the victory of Judah Maccabee and his sons over the Seleucids. Within a century, the Romans annihilated the Jewish state, exiled most Jews, and destroyed the Second Temple; Rome's arch portrays the capture of the Menorah. Rabbis argue that it was because of *Sinat Chinam* that the Jews weakened themselves. This is not the place to detail the raucous, even violent disagreements among the Jewish sectors. But recall the at times violent disagreements then:

- The Sadducees (*Tzedukim*) rejected oral Torah, denied afterlife and resurrection, and angels and belonged to the aristocratic priestly class;
- The Pharisees (*Perushim*), more the hoi paloi (common folk) accepted oral and written Torah, resurrection, angels, and afterlife;
- The Essenes were ascetic, withdrawn from society, lived communally, expected an apocalypse, and left us the Dead Sea Scrolls;
- The Zealots were militants against Roman rule;
- And we can include the Nazarene, early Christians who accepted Jesus as *Moshiach* (Messiah), who often practiced Jewish ritual (as did Christ and his disciples in his last Passover supper).

Certainly, we gather that each of these groups believed profoundly in their own sectarian version of Judaism, even self-righteously believed that they were saving Judaism from the other sectors. Were they not also behaving like Alter describes the otherwise well-meaning throngs of mostly secular Jews protesting the government's proposed laws to limit the Supreme Court? Further, much of the contemporary majority who voted for this government appeared to be from non-Ashkenazi or religious affiliation; this suggests that there were also "ethnic" contribution to the tension between our two contemporary groups. Ashkenazi (more secular) versus "Sephardi" and religious Jews who appear to be "taking over" the country.

To respond to Alter, whom I have found always, always thoughtful (and correct, especially about translation), our contemporary pre-October 7 "political" battlers were sincerely self-righteous as were the sects of two millennia ago. This is what I mean by *Sinat Chinam* today. What was missed (two millennia ago and today) was a common sense of being Jewish as a unifying principle. After all, Biblically, Joseph made a strategic decision to build a people and ultimately a nation from his scrabbling, contentious, even homicidal brothers. He could have just excluded the bad eggs. And Moses led *all* the surviving Jews to the promised land.

So, I return us to the addressing and resolving to overcome *Sinat Chinam*, in order to heal the torn souls after October 7. We need mending.

We cannot ignore, dismiss, and diminish the *mu'aka*, the deep distress, that the *Otef* families and communities face.[13] The war continues, not only in Hamas Gaza but also in Hezbollah's setting the North aflame. Not only the death threats from Iran but also supersonic (Iranian) rockets from far-off Yemen. And then there's Syria, Iran's way-station to Lebanon, a country held hostage by Hezbollah, or now by a former ISIS leader, that has murdered hundreds of thousands of fellow Arabs, gassed them to death. Imagine what the Syrians will do to their "enemies." Erdogan's Turkey now tries to join the fray against the Jewish State. This far-flung multination threat is amplified by Jew-hatred from Europe to Canada, from Australia to campuses of the United States, of course Russia and China. These are great geopolitical threats.

But much closer to the heart are the too many I met who knew those murdered on October 7, those kidnapped. On a Zoom get-acquainted meeting with a dozen or so psychiatrists and psychologists, S. introduces herself as a child psychiatrist, a mother of two from Kibbutz Erez, now evacuated to Kiryat Gat, and . . . whose father was murdered on October 7. How does one carry on a clinical focus after such an introduction? What can one say, unless resorting to the formulaic Orthodox, *zichrono l'vracha* (his memory may be a blessing)? It's a heart-stopper.

And there are the dynamics following October 7 that will resonate for better or worse. A., a labor and delivery nurse (mentioned in a previous chapter) is considered heroic for converting her kitchen table into a surgery ward. On the other hand, some wives demanded their husbands not go out to fight resulting in their husbands' guilt and those marriages may be faltering.

At night, even in Beersheva, the bombings can be heard from Gaza; and the whop-whop of helicopters evacuating critically wounded at day often by night. Dr. Meiri carries on running an entire child and adolescent psychiatry program, even as his mind is divided between one son in Gaza and the other poised at the Lebanese border. And, *and*, he tells the *kabanim*, the IDF psychiatrists and psychologists, what he hears from his son in Gaza is far more terrible than what he experienced in Lebanon or Tulqarm.[14]

Dr. S. is an example of someone who has been psychically paralyzed since October 7; she found the idea that shreds of her soul had been kidnapped, ripped from her, held hostage. But she realized that Hamas was not controlling this hostage; she had potential control. She is honest with herself that her children's education is better in their displaced Tel Aviv. She finds a way to return to her cottage in *Netiva Ha'Asara*, a way that her husband, a child of this Kibbutz who cannot bring himself to return. She has insight that will help reknit her family, recapture her "tribe" (*shevet*) and ultimately her community.

As a psychoanalyst, I favor internal work. Yet, as Natti Laor, a psychoanalyst/philosopher, has shown in his lifetime of work with traumatized communities, one must work with communities to rebuild them, after earthquakes (in Turkey) or Iraqi Scud bombings of Tel Aviv. Among many other innovations, he and colleagues introduced the concept of *chisun*, immunization as centers that can protect or strengthen the individual, the community, from traumata.

We can reflect on Erik Erikson's last book, in which he described families as built like engaged cogwheels; each generation a cog, engaging the others. Children engage parents, engage grandparents, and so on. Each moves the other and enriches the movement through life. This elegant, dynamic "mechanism," is evolutionary; it's built-in until something terribly goes awry, such as October 7. How to we repair this normative movement of generation to generation?

One hint is the quiet busyness that we found in the Kibbutz Erez preschool evacuated to Kiryat Gat. We would not have known while watching their rich, engaging play that these children had been evacuated, even that many had fathers, uncles, or older siblings at war in Gaza. Part of the secret sauce is the quiet, hovering attentiveness of the staff. The playful activities of music and movement, the free play outside with cast-off beaten-up kitchen utensils, and the rapidity with which the children engaged in creative drawing and storytelling. As mentioned in the children's chapter, it would be ameliorative (I avoid the overused word "therapeutic") for the parents of these children, the grandparents, even strangers like me, to spend a day or half-day weekly in this setting. Healing to watch the children, to play with them.

Part of the successful formula for the Kibbutz Erez preschool is the relatively close-knit community. People have chosen to live together in the Kibbutz; not just buy a house in the neighborhood, rather to share basic principles, that fit more under Weber's *Gemeinschaft*, felt, shared values. Kibbutzim have fallen out of favor in the last few decades. In fact, some Israelis considered kibbutzniks to be *fryers*, "suckers" for working a lifetime, yet never owning anything. But, as the Jewish-French poet/playwright, David Valayre has written, possessions, even our children, are like air that we breathe: only temporarily within us, even enliven us, yet must be released (albeit, like our exhales, transformed) into the world.

The previous *yishuv's milieu* (from the French, literally "mid-place" or within a matrix)—a significant weaving of *Gemeinschaft*, communality, commonality, even "brotherhood"—is amplified within the (few) Orthodox kibbutzim, such as *Alumim* (in the *Otef*) or *Kfar Etzion* (which I have known for over decades). Minimally, the residents are woven together at the daily (even two or three times daily) *shul* prayers. Deaths are a tear in the fabric that however can be rewoven. One needs at least ten to have a *minyan*, and a *minyan* is needed to read Torah or preferred to say Kaddish for the dead. Hence daily and for sure every Shabbat, there is an ingathering of residents before they disperse to fields or jobs elsewhere. And with the prayers come a way of living (613 commandments, although half can only be performed when the Temple is rebuilt). We will need to see how much the *datiyut* (religious belief) of the Orthodox *yishuvim* helps buffer them from this horror compared to the seculars. And not just buffer but recover. On the other hand, how can the Orthodox reconcile belief in a merciful God after the horror of October 7? We need to be patient and observe and learn from them.

But not only observe. We can facilitate practices to help the *yishuvim* recover and rebuild as communities, even as they mourn the tortured and murdered, as they continue to yearn for the hostages to be returned, as they worry about their sons and daughters in battle, as they worry about their own survival as Iran and its proxies try new ways to harass and kill Jews. Hence, any suggestions here are modest in the face of these ongoing challenges, *ha'mu'akot*, "the distress."

As with Oded Arbel's work with soldiers, *doing*, *building*, and *talking* are good combinations. He and their team "cleansed" their Zen-inspired communal room; ate together, played together and recounted the soul pains that they had heard during the day. The latter diminishes the impact of secondary traumatization, a less frequent theme addressed, for instance, in psychoanalytic literature, or rather, often discussed as (evoked) countertransference (Flarsheim, 1994).

The *yishuvim* could begin by jointly rebuilding structures, gardens, and furniture together, even before moving back. I think of the quiet, generous Amish from Australia living there for months, who paint and rebuild for the Kibbutz. (More recently, the Amish built small homes for the hurricane-ravaged North Carolinians, after our government's FEMA failed.) They are of German origin and I wondered if this was a form of repentance for what the Germans did to the Jews. I learned of a similar German Evangelical community in Northern Israel that has been there for decades: the members are dedicated to caring for the dwindling number of Shoah survivors.[15] But the 20-some-year-old blond-haired, blue-eyed daughter is serving in *Khilutz v'Hatzalah* (Search and Rescue) in the IDF: one of her two brothers was killed in the IDF service. There is a level of dedication that is extraordinary, even as they remain dedicated to Christ. She quoted a verse in Isaiah 40 for non-Jews (she believes):

"*Nachamu, Nachamu Ami,*" "Comfort, Comfort My People." Perhaps more will recognize this from Handel's *Messiah* (Sharratt, 2013).

Repair the Psyche; Repair the Community; (Am boneh Tzava, boneh Am)

I suggested to Sh. that the Kibbutz members might better be working side-by-side. Even the new fortress-like children's center might be built with kibbutznik parents and grandparents, even the children, working side-by-side with the professional bricklayers, carpenters.[16] Of course, they could be discussing the priorities of what needs to be reconstructed. What should be done with devastated often burned-out homes: keep as memorials; attempt to rebuild? I only suggest and then listen to their thoughts. Should all resources be spent first on a women's center (men and children excluded), or, well, or whatever else the community or its representatives prioritize? A question open for discussion.

Meetings will be complemented by "field interviews" as people go about daily lives (Redl and Wineman, 1965). But regular, scheduled meetings are productive, with the *yishuv* as a whole, broken into task groups, as Dr. Arbel has with his *Kaban* unit.

And Kibbutz security *will* change. I recall visiting Kibbutz *Re'em*, one of the older ones in the *Otef*; it was the tree from which branches were snipped and spliced to create sister settlements elsewhere, including *Be'eri*. We went to *Re'em* to "see" the members of Kibbutz Be'eri buried there temporarily; when *Be'eri* is habitable again, the rabbis have a ritual for disinterring the bones for reburial in *Be'eri*. (Ironic, that rabbis must bless this for members who are devout secularists. The Kibbutz member from *Re'em* read to us a secular substitute for the Kaddish written by a Kibbutz member some decades ago.)

As I said earlier describing him. This fiftyish *Re'em* kibbutznik wore his holstered gun, something he'd never done before. The Kibbutz will rethink locking their guns in an armory, something the Hamas terrorists knew about and hence hindered. This man was firm: while they still believe in the IDF, maybe in the local police, they will take their own responsibility for immediate responses to invasions.

We went to the *Be'eri* temporary *kevarim*, gravesites. In small groups, we gathered at different graves. It's customary to put a stone on someone's *kever* as an honor. But it felt unseemly to add the burden of even one more pebble, even one gram, to these lives; I placed a pebble next to each *kever*.[17] (I recalled Ben Gurion's burial site overlooking the desolate desert where the Israelites wandered for 40 years. Not a pebble adorned his *kever*, instead, stones were placed—hundreds—next to his, often between his and his dedicated wife's *kever*.) At each site, a guide spoke about who was buried there from October 7. At ours, Elhanon, our towering guide, a former history teacher, looking stooped as if shoulder-burdened by memories, spoke of each of the four members of the *Even* (Stone) family. The parents piled on their sons to protect them from the hail of bullets, to no avail. You'll recall, as one teenager was dying, he knew he was dying; he asked only that he be buried with his beloved surfboard. Which was done. In our imaginations, he remains perched on his board, riding Mediterranean waves; but he is no Greek Eros perched on a dolphin's back; he has been claimed by Thanatos. The father was a Jack-of-all-trades who would fix any mechanical thing on the Kibbutz . . . and if they were no longer reparable, would convert a tractor or backhoe into a multicolored sculpture for children to climb. I'm but a writer, a word-crafter: I have no words to describe standing before an entire annihilated family. No. Words. And no more stones would I burden this *Even/Stone* family.

I am also a physician: I have seen dying, I have seen death. I have seen nothing like this in my career. But, as a psychiatrist and child psychiatrist, I return to what we can do for the living.

Dr. Gal Meiri is establishing a child and family center in the *Otef*. This will have a new function, which we might call "post-vention": how to intervene now and for the future with all the children, triage of those who are more symptomatic; new mothers and how they are affected in ability connect with their babies, reading their feelings, for instance.[18] How to work with each *yishuv* to listen to the challenges of rebuilding: how many are returning; who are not and how do we help; how to mourn not only those who were murdered but also kidnapped and also those who cannot return. We met with the midwives of the South, who deliver all the newborns. We show them Bob Emde's 30 baby IFEEL photos, which assesses how accurately new mothers read facial expressions of babies. We think about how this is a way of screening those new mothers who are misreading babies; how to intervene early.

———

I know that Israel will both heal and build. Why? Because its most important natural resource is its people and its people are irrigated by and nourished by its eons-long culture as embodied in its Bible, in its stories, in its laws.

We can turn to Pericles' oration to understand the reason for optimism. When expected to give a funeral speech for fallen soldiers, Pericles demurred. Instead, he would first speak about the City-State of Athens and its inhabitants, for *this*, for *them* these men fought and fell. He continued:

> Our system of government (democracy) does not copy . . . our neighbors. It is a model to others . . . a democracy, because power is in the hands of the whole people.

And then he spoke of what he thought of as an asset, but after October 7, we might think of as also a vulnerability:

> Our city is open to the world and we have no periodical deportations in order to prevent people observing or finding out secrets which might be of military advantage to the enemy. (p. 179) . . . We rely on our own real courage and loyalty.

And he continues describing what could be also said of Israel and any great democracy at least since the Renaissance in Western Society:

Our love of what is beautiful does not lead to extravagance; our love of the things of the mind does not make us soft. We regard wealth as something to be properly used, rather than as something to boast about.

As for politics, he could be speaking of raucous Israel:[19]

we do not say that a man who takes no interest in politics is a man who minds his own business; we say that he has no business here at all.

(Thucydides, 1972, 94–99)

Pericles' funeral oration brings us to Lincoln's 271-word, ten-sentence Gettysburg Address. I cite it here, for two reasons. First, he says (ironically) "The world will little note, nor long remember what we say here, but it can never forget what they did here." Second, for our purposes, he alludes to healing the rift in the Civil War, brother against brother. He challenges the living to fulfill the unfinished work of the Republic, to honor the dead by living. Better, his words: "this nation, under God, shall have a new birth of freedom—and that government of the people, by the people, for the people, shall not perish."[20]

Lincoln returns us to our simultaneous task of healing *Sinat Chinam,* "brotherly hate." And the purpose: that "the people shall not perish."

When a Shoah survivor came to Rabbi Abraham Karp in Rochester, she complained bitterly about her "little" sister with whom she escaped, when 19 years old, from the Nazis to Soviet Russia and cared for her there. After the War, they learned that most of their remaining family were incinerated by the Nazis. The sisters married (on the same day, later gave birth on the same day), then immigrated to the United States aided by the Jewish Community. Since then, for decades, they had been scrabbling at each other's skin, opening old wounds, scraping psychic scabs, poisoning the minds of their own children against the other, refusing to meet except for the obligatory *seders* or for the children to play *dreidel.* They even joined different survivors' groups: one, proud of its "American" poker and card games, the other "too serious" for such things. She tried to enlist the good Rabbi on her side: tell her sister and explain why this older sister was in the right. And also, her Auschwitz-surviving brother was not right.

To which, Rabbi Karp responded with a tone of sadness, yet tenderness, something like this.

Hitler destroyed most of your family. By continuing to fight with each other, you give him an ongoing victory. A true victory for both of you is to respect the memories of those who died by not arguing, not fighting, not turning cousin against cousin.

The woman was my mother; her sister, and Auschwitz-survivor brother, my Tante Adele and her brother, Uncle Avram.

This is a "cure" for *Sinat Chinam*. We can use the idea of "soul-hostage" that many in Israel found useful. On October 7, terrorists murdered and tortured Israelis. Then they took hundreds hostage, some of whom remain hostage, all of whom suffered evil. But see how a part of your own soul has been ripped away and is now "hostage" to terrorists, to terrorism. This "hostage" is potentially in your control, can be liberated, and can be restored to you. Your repaired soul will not be like it was on October 6. But it can be whole. And it will be infused with the wisdom of how to live a full life.

The painful, cutting irony of *Sinat Chinam*, is that our "enemy" belongs to us, is our brothers and sisters; that in psychoanalytic terms, we project unto them unacceptable parts of ourselves, then attack them (and hence ourselves). To heal *Sinat Chinam*, we need to *focus on the common soul of the Jewish people*, not the minuscule narcissistic differences (Freud, 1930) that create chinks in our armor. Chinks that Iran/Hamas/Hezbollah/Whomever hope they could infiltrate and attack and destroy the Jewish people; not just a State but rather annihilate a people. We can turn to Virgil who counsels Danté, "put aside division of spirit/gather your soul against all cowardice." We must put aside division of the Jewish spirit, the Jewish people, and gather our souls to re-heal.

My initial perhaps odd title of this book was "From Hell to Eternity." There is a twist on meaning after writing (and rereading) this work. I intended to learn from Antique classical texts what "heroes" learned from having to go through hell, midway through their life journeys, midway through their return "home." But, reading the three classics, none contains the horrors of October 7.

Yet I realized that there is another meaning inherent in eternity for the Jewish people. We are an eternal people (insomuch as anything human can be "eternal"). Historically, we have endured for over three millennia as a people, as a culture, at times as a nation, and despite two millennia of exiles. Jews frustrated and dismayed the historian Spengler and Atkinson's thesis (1918/2021): other ("Western")[21] great cultures have risen, contributed to humankind, then fallen (Ancient Greece, Rome, Assyria, Egypt). Jews endure. Or at least, we have been long-lasting, as Bellow (2010) said of Sammler. In an odd sense, Jewish culture has been as enduring as three major Antique Asian cultures: Chinese, Japanese, and Indian cultures, cultures that have had the profound luxury of inhabiting their own lands, despite multiple colonial incursions—British (India and China), German (China), Japanese (vs. China), American (China and Japan), and the French (too numerous colonies to enumerate here).

The Bible states that we are created in the image of God; mimetic of God, we are, like the architect who built the temple, who designed it *betzelem Adonai*, in the shadow of God. In this very human sense, mimetically, we have an eternal being.

One of our cursed blessings is that we should be a "light" unto the nations. However, many Israelis would be quite satisfied lighting their own lives; leave other nations to themselves.

We are supposedly a chosen people, a questionable gift. When Abba Eban, then Foreign Minister had a highly secret meeting with an Arab Foreign minister (Saudi Arabia, I believe), the minister entered belligerently, refusing a handshake, demanding, "Who made *you* the chosen people!" Eban's response: "You want the job?"

But we can embrace our own eternalness: *we have been, we are, and we will be,* to echo God's answer to Moses when asked how he should be named for the Jews. We wish simply to be. And we will build ways to reestablish our lives, our nation, and our identities. We will repair the torn soul fragments, reunite our souls that *feel* held hostage (and reunite with human hostages remaining). Many others will learn from what we have achieved—another example of how Jews have contributed to humankind. But we do not exist for the sake of others. We need only remain eternal for our children and children's children forever, *l'olam.*

Fin

Notes

1 **Gemeinschaft** (based on affectional bonds) and **Gesellschaft** (based on rational, or mutual consent). Ferdinand in order to categorize social relationships into two types. The *Gesellschaft* is associated with modern society and rational self-interest, which weakens the traditional bonds of family and local community that typify the *Gemeinschaft.* Max Weber (1966) suggested a more fluid continuum between these states of social relationships. I thank my dear friend, Peter Friedman, a political scientist Z'L, for introducing me to these ideas via Weber as we jogged along the Chicago lakefront.

2 Shengold, was Oliver Sacks' psychoanalyst who, per Oliver Sacks, saved his amphetamine-addled life.

3 I use the old phrase to incorporate both acute stress and post-traumatic stress in soldiers. Note that Or's work in New Haven was with PTSD; today, we were discussing Acute Stress Disorder (or Reaction, as some military psychiatrists suggest we use).

4 Stockade and Wall was the determinant during the British occupation for a "legitimate" settlement. Hence, *chalutzim,* pioneers, would throw up a stockade and wall overnight to claim a new home.

5 For confidentiality, I omit the hotel's name.

6 The Kfar Etzion mothers and children, including Chanan, had been evacuated to Jerusalem before the attack.

7 She expressed concern in Hebrew to my host whether I could weather the steep climb. He responded, "He hits the gym daily."

8 I am excluding Sderot here, a larger city, but as it is divided into neighborhoods, like Beersheva, for instance, some of the ideas for repair may apply there also. I did not visit Sderot.

9 An example of such an American neighborhood is mine in Palo Alto, a very quiet, safe, wealthy town next to Stanford. In my cul-de-sac, when we moved in, one neighbor visited us with a bottle of decent wine, welcoming us, then telling us that they don't like to socialize and please do not visit them. Also, they were

protecting the squirrels of the cul-de-sac, and if our puppies endangered the squirrels, they would call animal control (which they did frequently) Another neighbor welcomed us, told us that he had just been appointed pastor of his Evangelical Church, that he once studied Hebrew, and that he would welcome saving our souls in the name of Christ. And our next-door neighbor, here for three decades, greeted us as our house had been recently painted by saying that she didn't like the color as it didn't match her house. We still had time to change the color, she said, and offered to advise us on picking a proper color. There was an overall tone of alienation in this very quiet, otherwise pleasant neighborhood.

10 This reminds me of my days in the ER at the University of Chicago on the Southside during the era of Black Panthers and such, when black-on-black gang fare was common, as was attacking and even killing U of C students and faculty. One early morning we received a 20-some-year-old gang member with a bullet wound through the heart. Technically, DOA. My resident, a chest surgeon, slashed open the ribs, shoved in his hands, found the entrance/exit wounds, plugged them, then ordered us to rush him to the OR. Some two dozen units of blood later, the fellow survived.

11 Although unlike the Romans, who I'm told only wanted fealty and taxes, the Iranian Shiites demand ruling one's inner life—or you will be murdered.

12 *Sinat Chinam*, from a psychoanalytic perspective, may be rooted at least in part in the primitive defense of projection: projecting onto others what one feels is undesirable in oneself. Then, one who does this feels "relieved" of unacceptable negative feelings and hence more self-righteous. Projection is a nefarious and destructive (of self and others) defense mechanism. Yet, even my esteemed Israel Psychoanalytic Society has not addressed the ongoing phenomenon in such psychoanalytic terms.

13 When I refer to the *Otef*, the envelope adhering to Gaza, I wish to extend it psychologically to those who are buffeted by the waves of October 7, at least in the Negev (and we know beyond). By beyond, I include not only October 7 but also the 350,000 reservists who flocked to fight and protect Israelis even by the next day.

14 On the other hand, I know Dr. Meiri to be a man of great modesty; he may be understating the horrors he too saw in those settings. But he reminds me of what the soldiers saw on October 7—babies incinerated alive, beheaded, women dead from rape, men whose faces or genitalia were shot off; these may be beyond what most soldiers have seen, even according to John Spencer, an expert in urban warfare.

15 For a powerful presentation by "Odelia," see https://www.youtube.com/watch?v=IFQKFwjwqmQ.

16 I recall the old kibbutz joke of a grandfather giving his grandson a tour: "My grandson, do you see this house, this road, this barn? I helped build it." To which the very modern grandson responds, "*Saba*, I didn't know you were an Arab."

17 I noticed later at Ben Gurion's *never*, overlooking the grayly, barren *Midbar Zin*, where the Jews once wandered for 40 years, that stones were placed next to, not upon, his *kever*. Also, on the path to his last modest home in *Sde Boker* was inscribed in stone a saying attributed to him, that a Jewish mother deserves a commander to oversee her soldier son, a Ro'i. A saying most poignant for October 7 and beyond.

18 Babies, for instance, have five distinct cries at birth; mothers know how to distinguish hunger from pain, from anger, and so on. Unless the mother has had adverse experiences. Using the IFEEL assessment, we can screen for mothers at risk for difficulties with their babies.

19 And we might add, he could be speaking of Elon Musk and his cadré, who engage in politics for the sake of democracy and free speech.

20 I give the full text here:

> Four score and seven years ago our fathers brought forth on this continent, a new nation, conceived in Liberty, and dedicated to the proposition that all men are created equal.
>
> Now we are engaged in a great civil war, testing whether that nation, or any nation so conceived and so dedicated, can long endure. We are met on a great battle-field of that war. We have come to dedicate a portion of that field, as a final resting place for those who here gave their lives that that nation might live. It is altogether fitting and proper that we should do this.
>
> But, in a larger sense, we can not dedicate—we can not consecrate—we can not hallow—this ground. The brave men, living and dead, who struggled here, have consecrated it, far above our poor power to add or detract. The world will little note, nor long remember what we say here, but it can never forget what they did here. It is for us the living, rather, to be dedicated here to the unfinished work which they who fought here have thus far so nobly advanced. It is rather for us to be here dedicated to the great task remaining before us—that from these honored dead we take increased devotion to that cause for which they gave the last full measure of devotion—that we here highly resolve that these dead shall not have died in vain—that this nation, under God, shall have a new birth of freedom—and that government of the people, by the people, for the people, shall not perish from the earth.
>
> (Lincoln, 1863).

21 My Israeli colleague Emanuel Berman questions my including the Greeks, the Romans, and, of course, the Hebrews among Western cultures. I do so insofar that they contributed to Western culture.

References

Aristotle. 1932. *The Politics*. Harvard (Loeb Library).

Bellow, S. 2010. *Mr Sammler's Planet*. Library of America.

Flarsheim, A. 1994. In Ed. P. Giovacchini, *Tactics and Techniques*, Volume 2, Jason Aronson.

Freud, S. 1930. *Civilization and Its Discontents*. p. 305. Hogarth Press.

Grinspan, Yossi, Elbaz, Shmeul, & Hadad, S. 2000. *K'she Halev Bocheh*.

Lévy, B.-H. 2024. *Israel Alone*, Tr. S. B. Kennedy. Wicked Son, an Imprint of Post Hill Press.

Lincoln, A. 1863, November 9. *Gettysburg Address Delivered at Gettysburg Pa. Nov. 19th, 1863. [n. p. n. d.]*. Library of Congress. https://www.loc.gov/resource/rbpe.24404500/?st=text

Redl, F., & Wineman, D. 1965. *Controls from Within*. Free Press.

Sharratt, Nicholas. 2013, Mar 21. "Comfort ye and Ev'ry valley" from Handel's Messiah. *YouTube*. https://www.youtube.com/watch?v=2Pz9BCMFoP8

Shengold, L. 1991. *Soul Murder: The Effects of Childhood Abuse and Deprivation* (1st Ballantine Books ed.). Fawcett Columbine.

Spengler, O., & Atkinson, C. F. 2021. *The Decline of the West*. Arktos.

Thucydides. 1972. *The History of the Peloponnesian War*. Penguin.

Weber, M. 1966. *The City* (1st Free Press Paperback ed.). The Free Press.

Weber, M., & Tribe, K. 2019. *Economy and Society: A New Translation*. Harvard University Press.

Index

For Product Safety Concerns and Information please contact our EU
representative GPSR@taylorandfrancis.com
Taylor & Francis Verlag GmbH, Kaufingerstraße 24, 80331 München, Germany

www.ingramcontent.com/pod-product-compliance
Lightning Source LLC
Chambersburg PA
CBHW070349270326
41926CB00017B/4053

9 7 8 1 0 4 1 0 1 7 2 2 6